Becoming Independently Healthy

Herbs of Grace

Other books by the author:

IRIDOLOGY
A complete guide to diagnosing through the iris and to related forms of treatment
(Thorsons – HarperCollins Publishers)

CREATIVE MENOPAUSE
Illuminating Women's Health & Spirituality
(Wisdome Press)

IRIDOLOGY COLORING BOOK
(Wisdome Press)

Becoming Independently Healthy

Herbs of Grace

Farida Sharan, MDMA ND MH

Wisdome Press
A Division of School of Natural Medicine
Boulder, Colorado

Wisdome Press
School of Natural Medicine
Post Office Box 7369
Boulder, Colorado 80306–7369, U.S.A.
Telephone/FAX (303) 443–4882

10 9 8 7 6 5 4 3 2 1

The author and the publisher are not responsible for your health, your disease or your journey on your own healing life path. We do not accept any responsibility for problems, adverse reactions or consequences resulting from the use of any remedy, suggestion, guidance, procedure or preparation included in *Herbs of Grace*. We wish you joy of healing on your journey.

Library of Congress Catalog Card Number: 94–076390

Sharan, Farida
Herbs of grace: becoming independently healthy / Farida Sharan.
p. cm.
ISBN 1–57093–003–1

1. Herbs–Therapeutic use. 2. Naturopathy. I. Title.

RS164.F37 1994 615'.321
QB194–780

Printed and bound in Boulder, Colorado in the United States of America.

This book is dedicated in love and appreciation
to my herbal friends and healers,
who gave me healing
and this new life
that supports my highest purpose.
Thank you.

Herbs saved my life when I was diagnosed with breast cancer and the doctor recommended a mastectomy. Herbs were waiting to help me even though I did not know anything about them. After creating healing and a new life, herbs formed the foundation of my work, writing, school, teaching and practice. Since then they have been my friends, and for twenty five years I have been learning about them, using them and integrating them into the complete system of natural medicine which is presented in this book.

I searched for a name that expresses the awe and gratitude I feel for the plant kingdom and what it offers us. During a summer vacation in 1978 I visited a village in southern France called *Dieu Le Fit*, meaning *God made it*. While I knew that was the message I wanted to inspire, there was no equivalent English translation. Then the name *Herbs of Grace* came to me. The image of divine grace healing humanity through herbs expresses my personal experience. Herbs radiate beauty, love and power. They make us stronger and healthier, ease pain and discomfort, relieve constitutional weakness and serve as our friends and helpers by offering inspiration, fragrance, beauty, food, medicine, useful products and abundant oxygen.

Acknowledgments

In May 1993 I woke up in my sister Thais's house in Vancouver, Canada, trembling and uplifted by a powerful dream. In the dream I was standing on ground that was encrusted with diamonds. Irregular patterns formed around the diamonds and then expanded into the universe where the diamonds became stars. Constellations formed from the stars and then condensed as they returned to earth where I was now standing on a giant patterned turtle with a diamond inside each design on the turtle's back.

I told the dream to my dear friend and student, Sandra, who is a member of the Turtle Clan. Shortly after I returned from a teaching trip to Australia and Malaysia in December 1993, I gave Sandra a black wood turtle from Bali to add to her collection. In February, after receiving a vision and painting for two days, she presented me with the painting 'Farida's Vision,' as a surprise, just when I needed a cover for Herbs of Grace. I give thanks for the love, the divine synchronicity and the beauty of Sandra giving such a magnificent gift to the book that she used for her own healing. This cover comes from our inner essence to explain the unexplainable through inspiration.

Herbs of Grace has been a work in process since 1976. For this paperback first edition, I offer my sincere gratitude to David Joel for his patient, caring and thoughtful editing which has helped me approach writing from a new level of conscious maturity. Thank you Sandra Patterson–Slaydon for your editing from the patient/student point of view. Great thanks to capable Michelle Steyskal and enthusiastic Tara Goldfarb–Elias, my bright and capable student assistants, who supported me through the whirlwind of creativity. Heartfelt thanks to my friend and graduate from Lebanon, Ghatfan Safi, whose beautiful iris drawings illustrate the Iridology chapter. A bountiful thank you to Carolyn Oakley whose willing support and humor made computer page design and formatting a fun adventure. Shawn Collins also offered computer support and willing rescue whenever we didn't know what to do – thank you! Superb proofreading from Richard Haight refined and polished the text. Bountiful thanks to Li Hertzi and Julie Noyes Long who created the cover design from my ideas. Deep appreciation to Carol Hotto for the index. The final proofing and editing that my daughter, Casel, did during the August 1994 summer school contributed the crowning touch. I also give special thanks to Anne Curtis, who patiently guided me through the world of printing in a supportive and caring way.

I have truly learned how much support is needed to create a book. I also want to thank the many patients and students who have written and telephoned over the years to share their appreciation for *Herbs of Grace* in its patient/pracitioner versions. This inspired me to publish this book, so that its truths and practical treatments may reach a wider audience.

About This Book

I offer this book from my heart and life, sharing my experience, my wisdom and my knowledge as a guiding light for others and a gift for the world. My cancer was cured and my life saved by applying the information I received from reading *Back to Eden* by Jethro Kloss. My work and this book are my way of expressing my gratitude for the new life these truths gave to me.

Throughout the book I advise you to work with skilled practitioners of the healing arts, to seek out the best health and healing teachers, to receive iris analysis, to educate yourself and to listen to your life with all of your being. This book was created and shared with the understanding that you will each take full responsibility for your life, your body and your health as I did. Each one of us is completely unique and each treatment must be applied correctly, sensitively and adjusted according to each moment in time.

This book presents a workable and proved system of natural medicine. While herbs are the core of the system, their use is guided by Iridology, the study of the iris of the eye, which is presented in the Iridology chapter. The other aspects of natural medicine, counseling, nutrition, flower essences and naturopathy, support and augment the use of herbs. As I expanded my experience of natural healing into these areas, seeing how their contribution supported the work of the herbs, I wove them into a complete and workable system, similar to systems which have existed in many ages and cultures.

Herbs work better when purification diets are used. There is no point in trying to go in two directions at once, so diet is adjusted to support the purification and rejuvenative influence of herbal nutrients. They also work better when poultices, baths, fomentations and enemas clear resistance and blockages. Students and graduates who have combined this system with orthodox medicine, nursing, homeopathy, acupuncture, and bodywork, all report the same truth, that their healing systems work better when they use herbs as nutrients, guided by Iridology, and supported and augmented by other natural treatments and purification or rejuvenative diets. Consistent success by hundreds of practitioners over nearly twenty years has proven the system that we present in this book.

Herbs are our teachers because they lead us towards healing. The more we work with them and the more we see them, love, touch, respect and thank them, the more they are able to help us. When we get to know them they also become our friends, and a relationship of love flows in exchange and gratitude as they teach us how to know and use them. When we use them internally and externally they make changes in our bodies that give us new life. There are many herbal books that explain what herbs do and how they do it, but the best knowledge is personal experience of their healing and the life energy that they give. Herbs become a part of us and create a vibratory resonance that increases our sacred connectedness with nature.

This complete herbal system is utilized within the energetics of purification, regeneration and transformation, processes of life which are death or degeneration, birth or creativity, and balance or maintenance that allows natural transformation. These exist dynamically in our life whether or not we are aware of them. When we are conscious of and cooperate with these processes, death and degeneration become purification, birth and creativity become regeneration, and the present moment as it unfolds naturally becomes transformation that supports our highest purpose. We allow our life to evolve without resistance and fear when we live in the present moment with trust, faith and surrender.

Every ecology is created of life/death/life cycles. Cycles of duality, night and day, winter and summer, death and life are in constant motion. We carry a fear of ultimate body death yet we know life continues all around us. If we live in the present we are born every moment. Our cells are dying and being born every moment of our existence. Our body completely renews itself every seven years. The more we cooperate with these energies the more we focus on the fullness of life and love in every moment. The death of our body becomes a letting go that allows the life of the spirit to open as we experience transformation in the present.

When we wish to harness healing energies we must focus not only on what is passing away but on the birth of every moment, as we learn to cooperate not only with creative energies of regeneration, but also with the dissolving energies of dissolution as we let old patterns go. By choice, we become the phoenix, dying and being born in every moment and using the nutrients of our ashes for renewal. To be truly alive we need the courage to live and die at every moment, to let old patterns and relationships pass away naturally and evolve into new forms which create space and nourish the new cycle.

After the general principles of this system of ancient and modern healing are presented in Health Ecology, the practical realities of the herbs are introduced in Herbal Instructions and Herbal Ecology. The next chapter on Nourishment guides us to use healing foods to support the herbs. After Herbal and Naturopathy Treatments, the Iridology chapter presents the basics of how we use iris analysis to guide the use of herbs and diet for healing as well as offering examples of the main iris signs and constitutional types. I share my mystical magical healing journey in the Healing Grace chapter to inspire those who are ready to walk this path of truth.

This book can be used effectively by several types of people. As well as being a workbook for clients, students and graduates of the School of Natural Medicine, it can be used as a reference by herbalists, iridologists, naturopaths and practitioners of other schools and systems of natural medicine as well as for lay practitioners who love herbs and healing. Many who use this book add to its visual display by coloring, pasting in pictures, highlighting and making notes. Enjoy this book as you make it part of your life.

Contents

DEDICATION 5

ACKNOWLEDGMENTS 7

ABOUT THIS BOOK 9

1 HEALTH ECOLOGY 13

Purification, Regeneration & Transformation 17

Purification 18

Regeneration 19

Transformation 21

2 ELEMENTAL ENERGETICS 23

The Five Elements 26

3 HERBAL INSTRUCTIONS 37

Create a Relationship With Herbs 38

Herbal Powders 39

Capsuling 40

Other Methods of Powder Preparation 40

Dosage 41

Herbs for Infants & Children 42

Herbs for the Elderly, Ill & Dying 43

Herbal Decoctions 44

Herbal Teas, Tisanes or Infusions 44

Herbal Tea Formulae 45

Individual Herbal Teas 46

Oils and Ointments 46

Baths, Footbaths & Handbaths 47

Tinctures 47

4 HERBAL ECOLOGY 49

5 NOURISHMENT 79

Breaking Addictions, Craving & Negative Food Habits 83
Fasting 86
Comfort Foods 87
Purification Diet 88
Mono Diet 89
Acid / Alkaline Balance 90
Liver Cleanse Drink 92

6 HERBAL & NATUROPATHY TREATMENTS 95

Abdominal Packs 96
Acute Illnesses & Accidents 97
Bath Therapies 100
Burn & Wound Paste 103
Candida & Yeast Infections 103
Castor Oil Packs 105
Enemas 106
Flower Remedies 112
Fomentations 115
Gall Bladder Cleanse 116
Healing Crisis or Achievement? 118
Herpes 120
Kidney/Gall Stone Cleanse 122
Kidney Ginger Poultice 123
Poultices 124
Prolapse Treatment 128
Referrals 129
Skin Care 131
Vaginal & Prostate Ovule 132

7 IRIDOLOGY & INNER ECOLOGY 135

Iris Fiber Structure – The Fabric of Life 136
Iris Structural Types 139

6 HEALING GRACE 165

APPENDICES 216

Nourishment Charts 207
Glossary of Iridology Terms 210

INDEX 211

1

Health Ecology

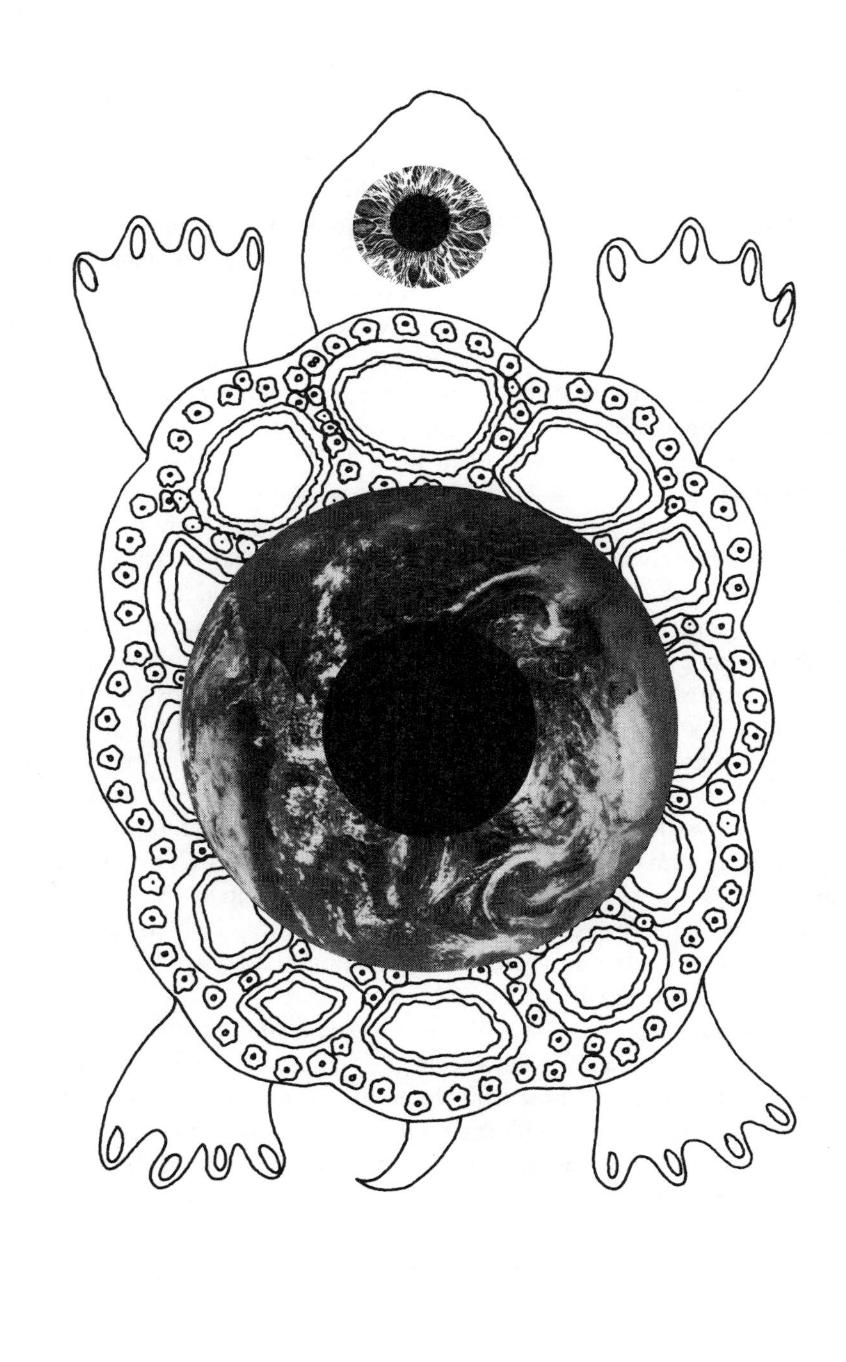

Health Ecology

Ecology is defined as the study of the relationships between living organisms and their environment. Most of us understand this concept and are familiar with ecological issues between human beings and today's world. However, it is important that we also become aware that we have a relationship with the ecological environment of our inner world. The outer world is affected by the inner world and the inner world is affected by the outer world. Both are affected by human spirit, mind, emotions, choices and the need for material products and nourishment. The more we realize the depth and importance of this truth, the more responsibility we will take for a respectful, considerate and caring relationship with both our inner and outer worlds. The more we live this truth, the more positive the effect we will have on our inner and outer worlds.

The ideal state of harmony in both outer and inner worlds is called *homeostasis*, which is the state of equilibrium within a living being that is achieved by positive healing forces that seek to compensate for any disruptive changes by adjusting and balancing. If we cooperate with these forces while seeking greater levels of health, well–being and healing, our inner ecology will receive the nourishment and support it needs to respond to and restore equilibrium of function, thus affecting all levels of our being – physical, emotional, mental and spiritual. As our inner world gains positive balance it will influence the outer world so that we can make a harmonious contribution to the world. We will give and receive nourishment from within and without.

Balance is achieved by harmonious dynamic interactions with several different energetics: body,/mind/ spirit dynamics, the relationship between the body organs, systems and glands and the forces of creativity, balance and dissolution, and our relationship with nourishment and the elements of life from which our body is formed.

Just as our outer world is made up of the elements of earth, water, fire, air and ether, we are also made up of the same elements. After we are born, the elements of our "world womb" become part of our inner world through digestion, breathing and skin absorption, which are all processes of metabolic transformation. These elements also exist in subtle forms in the emotions, mind and spirit and they are in a constant state of motion and change. As we evolve toward and enjoy balance with the elements, a state of equilibrium is achieved which supports our highest purpose and our spiritual life, offering us contentment, stillness and peace within the eye of the hurricane of constant change and disturbance which is life.

Inner ecology is supported or diminished by the quality of all our different relationships with the world – in the many and various realms of spirit, mind and emotions as well as by how we eat, drink, breathe and feel, how we give and receive love, nourishment, communication and service, and how we create and follow through with thought forms, goals, attitudes and desires.

Our bodies are woven of the elements of the outside world and require constant fresh supplies of nutrition containing all these elements. When we seek to restore health and accomplish healing, we gain the greatest results by nourishing the entire inner ecology, particularly the weak organs and systems simultaneously.

Our inner ecology is like an orchestra, and like the conductor we need to know how to bring out the best from each organ, gland and body system, so that we can understand how to make harmonious music within our body and life, in tune with divine harmony and the truths of life.

The relationship between our inner and outer worlds must be woven of respect which flows from love for our life and this creation. When we have that respect new relationships are formed with family, friends and society, with possessions, work and most importantly with our body and our inner world. We realize that this gift of life is precious. Our body becomes a treasure to nurture and heal. We tremble as we experience the sacredness of our being, and we bow our head in humility when we realize how we have created our own problems. Instead of focusing on shame, blame, guilt or anger, we choose to work with positive healing modalities and seek transformation.

When our body breaks down, there is a strong, clear message that we cannot live as we have in the past. Therefore the health challenge becomes an initiation. We can seek creative healing or we can allow the disease to run its course. Either way we have to move through a threshold, toward disease or toward health. When we choose health and creative alignment with the healing process, the path widens. A door opens. We sense a new future and a new potential. Love and gratitude awaken. Respect flows from our being. We have passed the initiation and our new level of emergence unfolds.

When we have a problem or when we feel threatened by ill health or death, we experience fear, heightened energy and a sense of urgency. The sacredness of the realties of life and death causes our hearts and souls to awaken. The intensity of living in this awakened reality supports our healing process because we discover and know ourselves on a deeper level. We have to understand why we needed this health challenge, what the disease is saying or doing that we cannot say or do. Through this process we become more powerful because we have realized a greater part of our potential.

When we become ill, normal boundaries and attitudes change. We realize our body and our life are ephemeral. We see how little control we have over events in our lives. Our concept of ego control falls away. We are forced to seek help and expand into a greater, wider vision. We seek true nourishment that gives healing and learn to let go of nourishment that is based only on stimulation, ignorance, taste, habit or indulgence.

The complete system of natural medicine based on the principles presented in *Herbs of Grace* offers an integrated, balanced treatment of herbs, dietary therapy and naturopathic treatments which help restore the balance of health ecology and establish deep and lasting healing. Treatment is guided by an iris analysis of the individual constitution and its inherent strengths and weaknesses. As the conductor of our own orchestra we need this information to create harmonious function.

How can we gain a deeper understanding of our inner health ecology? As described in the chapter Iridology, we use iris analysis to explore individual constitutional types, assess the function of the eliminative organs and systems, and to understand each individual's unique inner ecology. We also use iris analysis to educate people about their strengths and weaknesses and how their bodies will age or proceed toward illness. In–depth case histories reveal information about their life habits and dietary and nourishment imbalances. Consultations also reveal information about mental and emotional influences, as well as family, work and social stresses and strains.

Once a clear and full picture of all the aspects of a client's inner and outer worlds is obtained and explained, a program is created which includes herbal nutrients, dietary changes and treatments to cleanse the body, activate all the eliminative channels, strengthen weak areas, and balance the ecology of all the systems and organs. We recommend herbs guided by Iridology because this is a holistic way of balancing the inner ecology. We have proved again and again with students and clients that when all the weak areas of the body are treated simultaneously, the effect is better and longer lasting than if only one or two organs or systems which have surfaced as symptoms are treated at one time. It is essential to adjust the entire ecological balance of the body when treating any areas of weakness or symptoms.

Skilled practitioners make this health ecology educational process easier and quicker because they are able to gather and present the information in a fresh way, educate the client about what Iridology reveals, show the causes of the symptom picture and present a healing program which can be accepted and understood on a deep level. Because the information is fully explained, the client can make a commitment to create health and healing.

It is essential that clients understand that a minimum of three months is required to begin or make health changes, with a commitment to a longer program if necessary for release of chronic patterns, or if the client is not able to put into practice the full program. Each client's unfolding is individual and depends on many factors such as age, life habits, stress, shock, constitutional type, the effect of poor living habits over varying lengths of time, available support, personality, work and family responsibilities and so on. After three months clients decide whether they are satisfied with current progress and wish to terminate the treatment, whether they want to continue and achieve a deeper level of progress, or whether this program is something they will dedicate themselves to regularly whenever stress and life challenges lower their ability to maintain normal health.

Clients graduate as students of their own bodies, lives and inner and outer ecologies.They take away valuable information and tools for living, for tuning into their body, mind and spirit dynamics, and for recognizing when disharmonious life experiences have stimulated breakdown in normal body functions. They are guided toward restorative practices which will prove themselves by their results and which are helpful during further health crises. '*Know Thyself*' and '*Heal Thyself*' are the goals of this system of natural medicine.

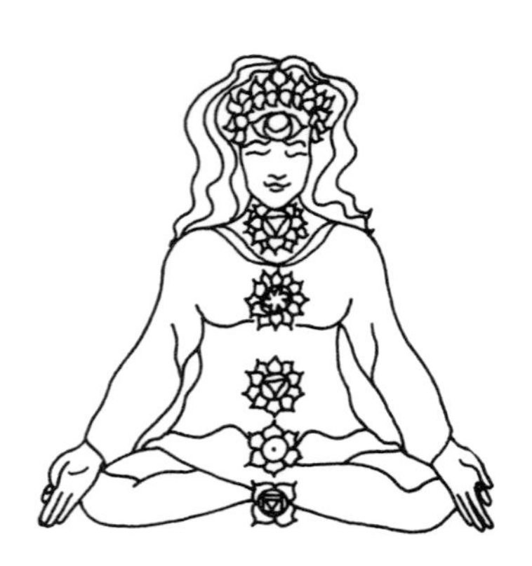

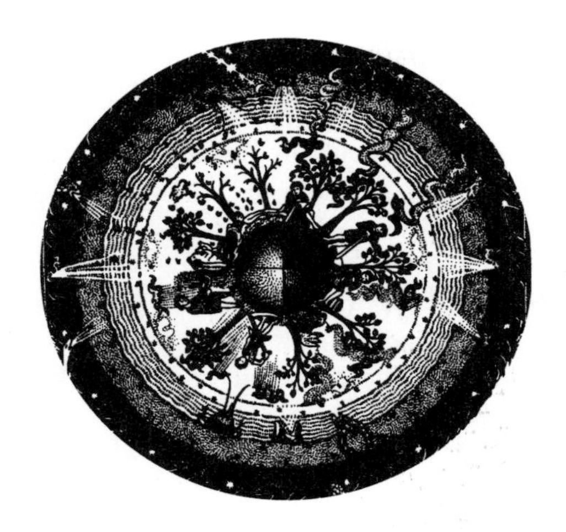

Purification, Regeneration & Transformation

The principles of purification, regeneration and transformation constitute the healing life dynamic which is the basis of this system of natural medicine. Movement or transformation is created in the life of the individual as toxins are eliminated on all levels, creating space which can be filled consciously with positive, loving, regenerative, physical, emotional, mental and spiritual nourishment. As a higher vibratory rate is achieved, the person's life opens and flowers into the next level of emergence. When nourishment is given lovingly to the body on a daily basis, the individual can seek other forms of nourishment in creative, emotional, social, mental and spiritual realms. The higher self can explore, seek and receive nourishment because it knows that basic levels are being taken care of in a responsible way.

The key to integrating and utilizing this complete system of natural medicine is to understand that the principles of purification, regeneration and transformation release one from imprisonment in their Gordian knot disease pattern. Whenever the interior ecology has been disrupted, and symptoms of fatigue, inflammation, toxicity, pain and discomfort and their accompanying negative mental and emotional states have become daily experience, the disease pattern has to be cut. It cannot be untangled because it is too complicated. The mental, emotional and physical threads which wove this life pattern have to be cut by an internal decision, commitment, detachment, completion and willingness to let go. The positive movement out of mental and emotional stress and conflict is augmented by the use of Bach flower remedies and counseling together with a natural healing program which includes a complete change of daily living habits, foods and beverages.

Once the new program is created and set into action, changes begin immediately. Each fresh cause that we make for health will ripen and bear fruit. The more causes we make, the greater the harvest of health. As the new patterns are lived on a daily basis, the old patterns lose their strength. Through the continuum of day–to–day choices new cause and effect patterns create a positive future because of freedom from the past and action in the present. New habits reverse the downward spiral of negative influences on the inner ecology.

PURIFICATION

Purification is the primary principle of the healing continuum. Most people today know that they carry a level of toxicity in their physical bodies, as well as mental and emotional toxins which help create physical blockages and malfunctions. The earth's air, water and soil are polluted. Most of our foods and drinks contain added chemicals, preservatives and dyes. The stress of emotional and mental conflicts in personal, family, social and work arenas confuses our abilities to digest and assimilate nutrients, alters body chemistry and changes food into poison. Stress and anxiety as well as emotional excesses cause the nervous system to secrete excess acids into the body, adding further to the burden.

When toxins become irritating and fatiguing factors within the body, the prime goal of an individual's three month program is to activate elimination and increase the release of toxins from the body so that daily elimination returns to normal. This activation, when guided by Iridology, proceeds in a gentle, balanced manner because the individual organs of elimination are stimulated on a daily basis.

During an iris analysis, practitioners usually discover that two or more of the eliminative channels are underfunctioning, and that perhaps one or two are compensating by over–functioning. Restoring and maintaining a balanced and active elimination is essential to good health and a balanced inner ecology. The increased life harmony and energy experienced when this is achieved speaks for itself. Clients return to the state of well–being they enjoyed when their body functioned naturally, without drawing attention to specific areas with symptoms, fatigue and distress.

When toxic release is allowed, the letting go achieves purification and creates space. When space exists, receptivity to new patterns is greater. The elimination of the old, creates a welcome for the new. There is an opportunity to establish new patterns, build new cells and create a new life. However, it is essential to prepare for purification and release. Forced or excessive purification creates unnecessary reactions.

Some people accept change, others resist it with every fiber of their being. For others, weakness, responsibilities or age make it necessary to facilitate a slow period of transition. Clients need to approach life changes from their unique personalities and their particular place in their life continuum. Practitioners must avoid processing everyone from one point of view.

This system of natural medicine is effective because it is guided by constitutional, physical and psychological models of Iridology. Therefore, each relationship is unique, treatment programs are individual, and transitions are given personal attention.

Herbal and nutritional programs support a gentle transition and avoid unnecessary healing crises and reactions. Each client is guided when discomfort occurs and is taught how to adjust the treatment or weather the discomfort utilizing natural therapeutic means. This serves as a teaching guide for the future. Eventually clients learn to listen to their body messages and know exactly what to do. Clients graduate and no longer require the assistance of the practitioner. The course of study and treatment is successful only when clients become independently healthy.

Purification must be approached carefully and slowly. For instance, whenever specific treatments such as liver, gall bladder or kidney cleanses are administered, the body should be prepared with applications of poultices, packs, massage, baths and enemas. Specific areas are relaxed, softened and defused before the cleanses are applied.

It is best not to go on an intense fast immediately, however potent the result of such a fast could be in terms of elimination. Fasting is not always necessary, nor is it always the best solution. It is not wise to go on a fast before all the eliminative channels are active. Also, fasts must be preceded by herbs and preparatory diets. Mono and purification diets or juice fasts often obtain the desired results in a gentle way, allowing clients to go about their daily life with relative ease. This is why applying the complete system of natural medicine is so important. It approaches healing through balancing and integrative processes. No one organ, system or gland is treated individually. All body areas are brought into harmony and to increased levels of function and strength so that imbalances do not occur.

It is also essential that eliminative methods do not purge the system, causing weakness and flooding the blood and lymph with poisons. This system of natural medicine creates a balanced, gentle approach which takes place while clients continue their daily life duties and responsibilities. Each aspect of the process, whether herbs, diet, life habits, flower remedies or counseling, supports the other aspects so that the movement of the continuum toward health avoids uncomfortable and debilitating healing crises.

Occasionally minor discomforts may appear. Clients may need to curtail unnecessary social engagements to conserve energy and utilize time and focus for healing. They may also need to seek advice to adjust the treatment. However, for the most part the process uplifts and improves health and well–being even as the treatment progresses. Any reaction is utilized as an opportunity to apply natural therapeutics and is approached as an educational opportunity. The body is teaching us lessons and we learn to listen and take appropriate action before negative conditions develop.

As so many symptoms disappear during purification, this system of natural medicine does not focus on any individual symptom or name of disease. The body, emotions, mind, and spirit are altered at a deep level. Strengthening of constitutional and eliminative weaknesses brings the body back to normal function, eliminating the cause of the symptoms.

Regeneration

Regeneration takes place at the same time as purification. Nutrients are provided by appropriate diets and herbs to support, regenerate and strengthen areas of weakness or deficiency. As old cells are eliminated new cells are formed. Herbs offer superior nutrition for specific glands, organs and body systems and areas. They are blended to feed every part of the body that is deficient – activating, cleansing, supporting, strengthening, rebuilding and harmonizing the inner ecology of the body.

The Nourishment chapter offers dietary therapies which support the work of the herbs so that the person is not going in two directions at once. Evaluation of the digestive processes is essential to guiding any program. How do people eat? Do they eat too fast? Do they chew well? Do they drink with their meals, diluting saliva and cooling the stomach with ice water? How do they combine foods? Do they eat junk foods? How many times a day do their bowels move? How much liquid do they drink in a day and what kind? How do they turn food into poison? What tastes do they crave? What foods upset them or cause allergies? What do they eat and drink all through every day? It takes a detective's mind to uncover the truth about nourishment patterns as well as the skills to educate the client and organize an effective individual healing program.

The emotional climate during eating and drinking must also be considered. This can include dysfunctional family relationships, stress and poverty in the past or present. Do clients eat while making difficult business deals? Do they have addictions, anorexia, bolemia, indulgences or cravings? Food and drink imbalances all reflect the wider aspect of their relationship to nourishment. Exploration and healing of these unnatural tendencies are an essential part of the healing process. How individuals receive and use nourishment reveals a deeper aspect of their approach to life and the causes of their health problems. Do they hold on to what is no longer good for them? Do they eat but still feel hungry? In what form does starvation and lack of satisfaction become constellated around food and drink? What nourishment are they missing and seeking? How are they using food and drink to deny or substitute real nourishment?

Food can be poison. Food can be medicine. Food can also be just food. When we create poison out of food it is as though we are purposefully cooperating with destructive processes. There is a short circuit of denial between what we do and the effect it creates. It is as though we have forgotten cause and effect. These factors must be discovered and brought into the light. We must be willing to create a nourishment pattern that will not only heal but also maintain health.

It is important to realize that the healing process should not be extreme and that it is not necessarily accompanied by acute fevers and crises. These reactions may occur when life threatening situations or severely chronic diseases require more powerful, drastic courses of treatment. Such advanced states of illness require full–time care in recognized, established institutions, such as the Gerson Cancer Clinic in America, or the Bristol Cancer Clinic in England.

The building of conscious health is the goal of this system of natural medicine. The focus of treatment is on eliminating toxins, creating space and rebuilding the body with rejuvenating foods and nutrients. A clean, well functioning body will not tolerate disease. It will adjust the symptom picture naturally as it returns to normal harmonious function, increased energy and higher fluid and tissue integrity.

The concept of homeostasis, or balanced interior ecology, where all aspects of body functions are neither overfunctioning nor underfunctioning, and where health is a natural, normal state of being, where all parts of the body are doing their work, is the key to understanding this system of natural medicine.

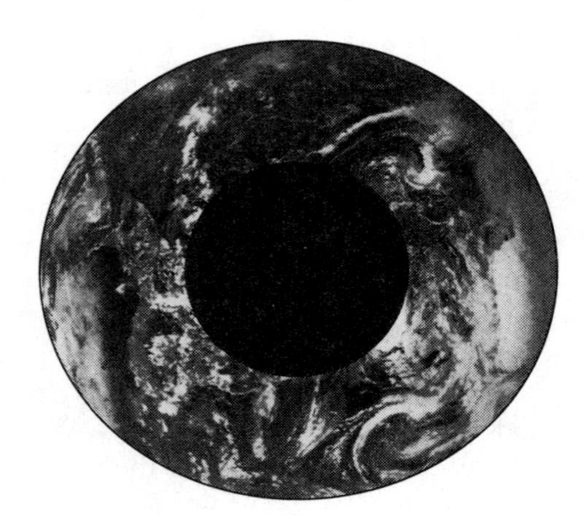

TRANSFORMATION

Transformation occurs naturally when toxins are released. Space is created which allows us to welcome the next level of emergence. If there is a desire for transformation, this will occur more easily when the body is purified, nourished, balanced and the inner ecology restored to harmony.

Transformation occurs when you live in the present, neither holding on to the past nor living in the future. When you are fully present without being burdened by the past or lured by the future, you can cooperate consciously with the possibilities for learning and evolution that are present in every moment.

We need to prepare for a new level of emergence. When old patterns are left behind, opportunity is created to choose new patterns. Vibratory affinities lead us in new directions. Old jobs, friends and patterns fall away naturally and are replaced by the new. Change flows more easily. Fear and resistance diminish. Trust and enthusiasm awaken childlike exploration. Instead of our life presenting us with resistance and with guardians at every gate that repeat one message, "Go within and do your work before you seek the next level," the universe opens before us once again with ease and joy.

The healing process itself means giving love, attention and nourishment to oneself. One's own being and body become the priority and therefore increase in value. This process of loving and caring for your body and life continues into the new cycle. Instead of ignoring or sacrificing ourselves to achieve material goals, we create a new balance between ourselves and our inner and outer worlds. We learn to say yes or no from a grounded perception of worth, balance and priorities. We realize that the choices we make from moment to moment create our future and we take greater care to make choices that take us where we want to go. The journey of our life within our body through this world is the most interesting and fascinating journey we will ever take. I invite you to enjoy the mystery and the journey.

What is transformation? *Collins English Dictionary* defines it as a radical change or alteration. In other words, a turnabout. What was before is no more. Like snakes, we shed our skins. Like snails, we leave our shells behind. Letting go is the first step. The second step is adding the new. The result is transformation. New causes create a new future. Our life opens up before us once again. Movement is life. Movement is transformation. Life becomes day–to–day, moment–to–moment transformation.

Living in the present means living from your growing edge. Being fully alive in the present allows you to live transformation in a mutable mercurial continuum. Each day is different. Ease and relaxation occur naturally as energy is released from holding on to the past or anticipating the future. The need for projection or anxiety passes away. Instead of tensing against change we relax and flow into it. We dance with the universe, unfolding the flower that is our soul.

So many people want to be different, better, healthier or more successful than they are. They have an idea of a better version of themselves that never manifests, that keeps them unsatisfied. Yet they do not do what will create that person. Often they do the opposite. These dreams and fantasies do not materialize because they do not stay in the present with choices. Instead of making choices consciously and saying "This choice will get me where I want to go," they say, "Because I am not what I wish to be I will have this pleasure to make me feel better." Substitution, instead of transformation, becomes a way of life .

We have many possible selves and yet most people get stuck in one version. They do not try different lifestyles easily, or explore, create, change or risk. They cling to what is familiar, yet long to be different. Transformation is about dreams becoming real, about people becoming who they want to become, about being successful in the way they want to be successful, about realizing their highest goals.

Transformation happens naturally as a part of the healing process. Often it happens in completely unexpected ways, as with my own story which I share in the chapter Healing Grace. I never imagined that an international school would grow out of my healing, that I would have a successful practice, teach, write books and travel worldwide. My new life unfolded as I made new choices and changes. My life became filled with purpose. Constant transformation and a life that allows time and energy for that process, is now my way of life. Outer duties and responsibilities are adjusted according to the time and space needed for my inner evolution. For me, a life of transformation equals freedom, because I am continuously moving forward on my life journey with joy and creativity. Time is available for what is truly important.

Transformation is individual and directly related to one's unique life experience. What transformation means to one person will not be the same for another. Each person will discover what transformation means for themselves by experiencing it as a part of their creative living and healing process.

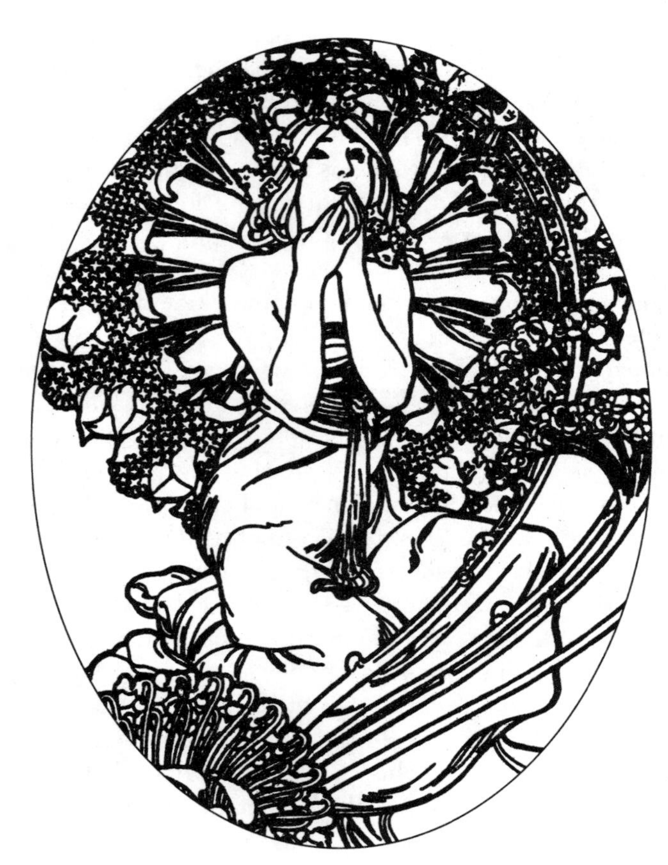

2

Elemental Energetics

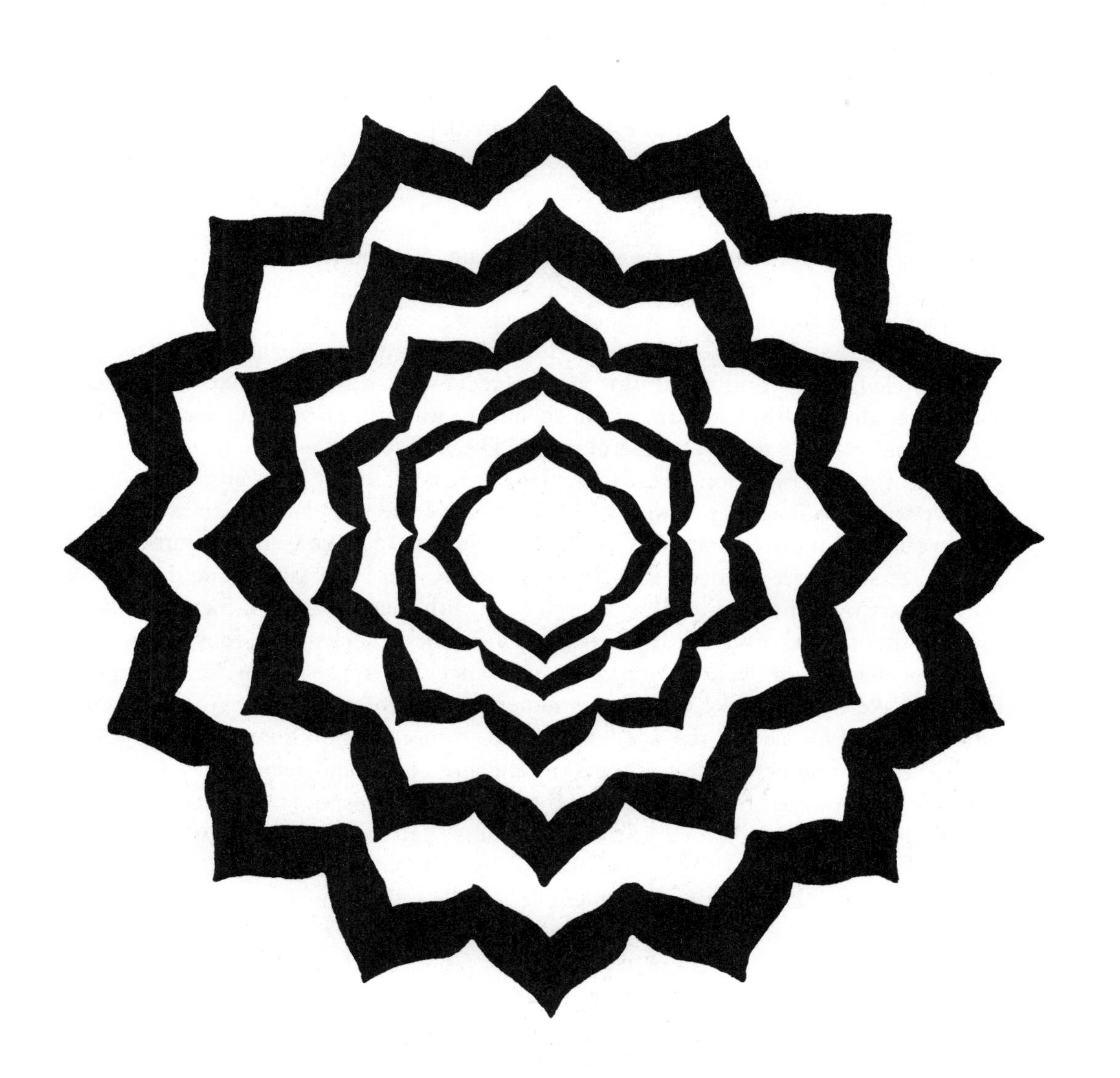

Elemental Energetics

"If you don't dance the elements, they dance you."

Like the child in the mother's womb, we are dependent on nature in an intimate, symbiotic relationship. Our intricate ecological alchemy requires the stimulation, energy and nutrients we receive from our elemental universe, as well as the more subtle nourishment from mental activities, emotional relationships, and spiritual grace. Our choice of nourishment determines the harmony or disharmony, consciousness or unconsciousness, wisdom or ignorance, which forms the foundation for our experience of our inner and outer worlds.

Our bodies and our inner and outer worlds are woven of the elements of life – earth, water, fire, air and ether. We are created from these elements within our mother's womb and are born into the elemental world womb. In order to receive nourishment from the elements of earth, water, fire, air and ether, and transform them into warmth, energy and nutrients, we eat, drink, breathe and absorb warmth, light and prana. The nature that sustains us in the outside world is processed through digestion, breathing, glandular response and skin absorption into active and subtle energies in our interior world. This mystery of the elements is woven into and contained within our body for the duration of our life. I invite you to make your life journey more conscious and to become aware of the elemental energetics in your body, your life and your world. As you gain mastery over them you will be able to work with them, play with them and be nourished by them, without being driven by them. If you don't dance the elements, they dance you.

The elements of life need to be kept in balance. Just as the conductor of an orchestra knows how to make the most out of each instrument and harmonize them in relationship with each other, we need to become the conductor of our own elemental life orchestra. Most of the time our bodies run haphazardly because we are unconscious of the elements, their purpose and their dynamic action in our lives. However, we can create harmonious music and movement with our bodies and our lives. We can attune our personal elemental vibration with the divine harmonious resonance in the cosmos, and live awakened elemental truths. The vibratory frequencies associated with each element create the full resonance of elemental harmony. Each element must ebb and flow, nourish the other elements, and make its contribution to the masterpiece of our lives in creative motion. When blockages, shortages or excesses create elemental disharmony, we suffer mentally, emotionally and physically. If we want to become our own conductor we need information. This system of natural medicine inspires individuals to adjust to the constantly transforming cosmic forces working within their lives. The more we participate in self–discovery the wider the horizon and the more limitless the possibilities.

Elemental Colors

The colors and energies of the elements flow down from the turquoise throat center where the goddess, Iris, expands the rainbow colors of green, yellow, orange and red into the world.

From this etheric emptiness, vibrations of sound and light that affect both our individual microcosm and the infinite macrocosm are given and received. We can use colors for therapeutic healing of imbalances and blockages in our physical, emotional or mental elemental energies and in our daily lives to expand our possibilities. If we prefer or avoid one color this reveals valuable information for our healing process.

Elemental Emotions

Excesses or shortages of any of the elements produce imbalances in our emotional life. Unbounded or frozen passions create a ground of disturbance which invites physical problems. The use of flower essences, emotional and mental therapy, and bodywork, combined with meditation and spiritual evolution, can help us tame and balance emotions so that we can rise to the grace of sensitive feeling, higher mind, spiritual compassion, tolerance and unconditional love that is not disturbed by the negative aspects of the five elements.

Elemental Medicine

The elements of life have been a valued part of every system of medicine in every age and part of the world, except in modern day orthodox medicine. The mystical and yogic systems of India and Tibet describe the elemental centers as 'chakras,' or wheels of energy that correlate to the physical endocrine glands and nerve plexuses. Each of the chakras relates to one of the elements of earth, water, fire, air and ether. In the Chinese system a slightly different organization of the elements is related to the meridians. The ancient Greek, Roman and Islamic systems describe the elements as humors. The forces of nature are feared, revered, respected and placated by primitive peoples who recognize our intimate relationship with the elements.

The elements can also be recognized in foods, herbs, climates, treatments and many other aspects of life. The elemental energies contained in all these different influences can create illness if misused, or help bring about a return to health when they are used therapeutically.

Imbalances of the elements create disease because of excess energy and irritation, or lack of energy and deprivation. Health is created from the balanced interaction of the inner ecology of body systems, organs and glands interacting harmoniously with our emotional, mental and spiritual bodies, and the world we live in.

The Elements and Mystical, Spiritual and Religious Experience

Mystical spiritual paths teach us that the worldly elements reflect the true elements of the spiritual regions. We learn that the elements of this world are transitory, mutable, transforming, nourishing, powerful and seductive. When we bring them into balance we receive the gifts and positive energies of each of the elements. However, we must strengthen ourselves or they may also challenge or tempt us. When in balance the elements nourish our spiritual journey and cooperate in the return of earth, water, fire and air to the ether element, so that contentment, peace and stillness supports our spiritual practice and our highest purpose.

When the spirit leaves the body during the death transition, all the elements return to their source: earth to earth, water to water, fire to fire, air to air and ether to ether. They are released from their bondage to each other which held body, mind and soul together for our lifetime.

The Earth Element

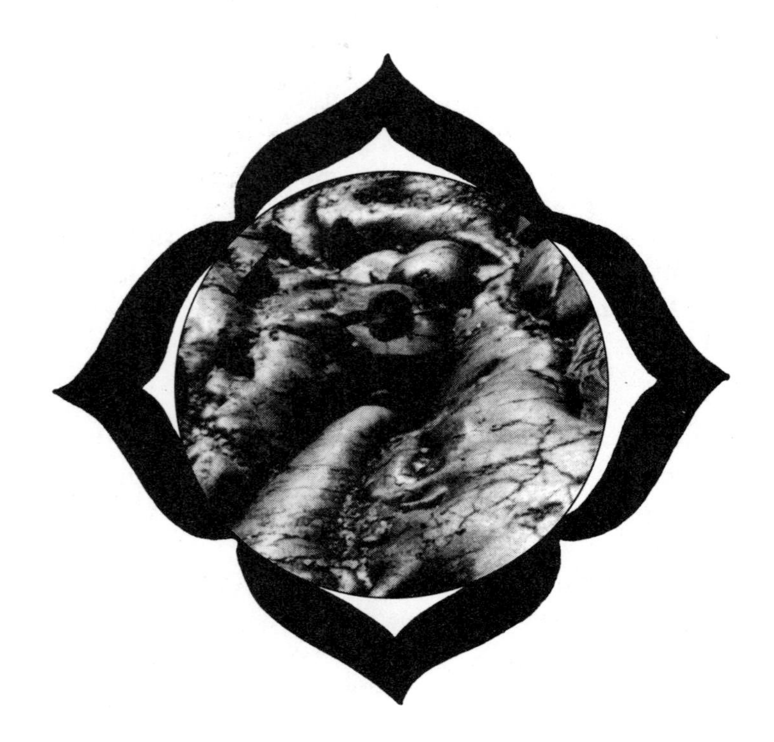

Chakra	Four petal Muladhara root chakra
Earth body location	Bones, sacrum, coccyx, adrenals, sciatic nerve, legs, perineum, large intestines
Earth dynamic	Yang, masculine, active
Earth color	Red
Earth emotion	Fear, panic, terror, anxiety, worry
Earth sense	Smell
Earth taste	Sweet
Earth astrology	Capricorn in the knees; Virgo in the stomach; Taurus in the neck

Earth energetics

Inert, downward, resistant, heavy, limiting, structural, supportive, hardening, dense, still, constant, solid, stable, inert, grounding, disciplined, crystallizing.

Earth lessons

Manifestation, grounding, limitation.

Positive earth energy

Abundance, security, prosperity, strength, health; respect for and the ability to work with and manifest from grounded structure and limitation by honoring practical laws.

Negative earth energy

Fear and clinging to security, possessions, land, home and body; afraid to risk.

Earth healing

Desert, mountain, rocks, sand, mud, caves, minerals, nutrients, grounding and the release of tension, stress and static electricity through contact with the earth.

Earth challenge

Survival without rigidity. After the basic needs of hunger, rest, warmth and shelter are taken care of, we protect our self, family, home, land and country.

Earth element emotions

Fear has many faces and can affect our lives in many ways: as insecurity, panic, terror, anxiety about known and unknown things and worry. Some people overcompensate and invest in material security, but sacrifice spontaneity and the rewards of risk. Others may talk themselves out of doing anything because they fear the worst, and thus miss opportunities. Worry and anxiety take away the joy of the present moment because we waste our energies imagining things that rarely happen.

Earth element disease

A shortage of the earth element creates bone weakness, adrenal problems, shaking and an inability to maintain balance or to walk. An excess of the earth element manifests physically as gall stones, kidney stones, constipation, hardening of the arteries, spine and bone problems, sciatica, muscle tension, and tight fists that won't let go either to give or receive.

The Water Element

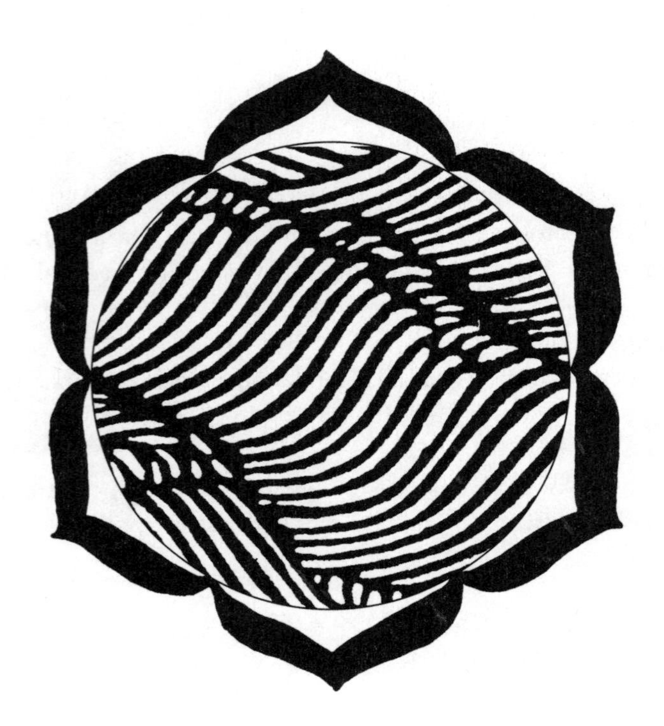

Chakra	Six petal Svadhisthana sweetness chakra
Water body location	Reproductive and urinary organs and glands; fluids
Water dynamic	Yin, feminine, receptive
Water color	Orange
Water emotion	Desire, repulsion, attachment
Water sense	Taste
Water taste	Salty
Water astrology	Pisces in the ankles; Scorpio in the genitals; Cancer in the breasts

Water energetics

Movement toward or away from someone or something, based on attraction or repulsion, which creates wave motions and a pendulum effect of action and reaction.

Water lessons

Consuming or obsessive desires must be disciplined as we consider the effect of our actions on others. Although it is important to let go of inappropriate desires, we must not suppress, repress or deny our feelings either. If we flow with the water, we learn to adapt and adjust and take the path of least resistance.

Positive water energy

Loving sexuality protected by social structures; true expression of deep feelings; natural grace and flexibility; the ability to nurture others with touch, warmth, understanding and love.

Negative water energy

Lust which sweeps aside the needs of others, ignores social boundaries and is never satisfied; or the frozen lack of emotion caused by repression, suppression and denial.

Water healing

Baths, steams, sea water, tea, sprays, douches, enemas, showers and waterfalls that utilize the cleansing, dissolving qualities of water to liquify, soften and release.

Water challenge

Move beyond the emotions of desire into the grace of deep feeling, instinctual knowing, and stillness that lies beyond personal attachment.

Water elemental emotions

Attachment is woven from desire, lust and possession of what pleases or satisfies, and rejection of what does not please or satisfy. It is also formed from our projections, desires, and human personal needs for sexuality, nurturing and giving and receiving love. Traditional social structures protect relationships through family and community bonds. Many people experience only the superficial emotions of attraction and repulsion, and the changeable moods associated with those dynamics. When positive and evolved, deep feeling and instinct reigns, and truth supports life's highest purpose.

Water element disease

Excess of the water element causes water retention, perspiration, and urine malfunctions, and the need for constant drinking. Shortage of the water element causes dryness, thinness, lack of perspiration, scanty urine, lack of thirst and resistance to bathing and drinking.

The Fire Element

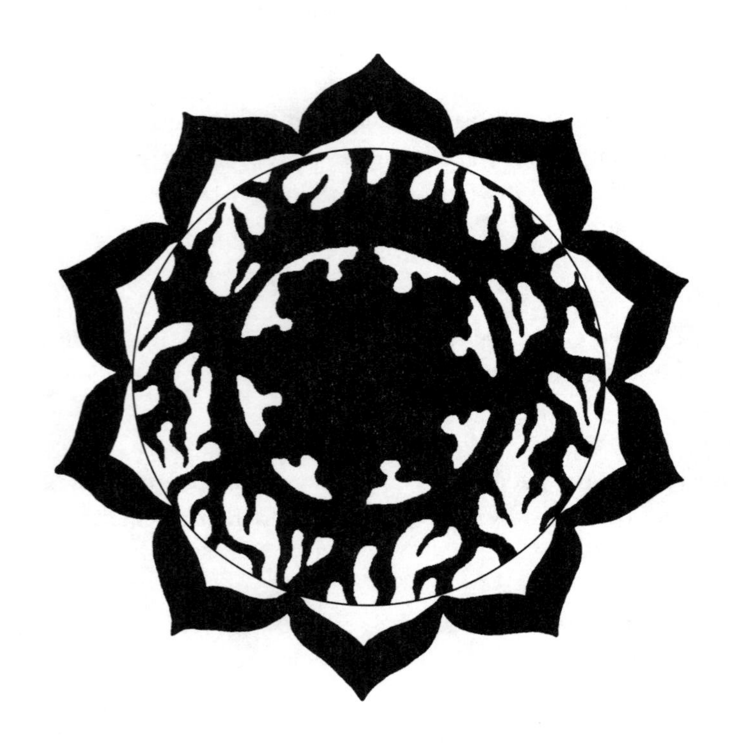

Chakra	Ten petal Manipura lustrous gem chakra
Fire body location	Digestive organs
Fire dynamic	Yang, masculine, active
Fire color	Yellow
Fire emotion	Anger
Fire sense	Sight
Fire taste	Pungent
Fire astrology	Sagittarius in the thighs; Leo in the solar plexus; Aries in the eyes

Fire energetics

Overcomes inertia; moves upward and transforms raw material through combustion into energy, power, light and warmth.

Fire lessons

Personal will must not be inconsiderate, manipulative, abusive or selfish. We must learn to align our personal will with the divine will so that we do not sacrifice the best of life to power struggles. Although we seek transformation and change we do not need to harm others with anger and destruction.

Positive fire energy

Energy for transformation; healthy digestion; excellent sight; willpower and the ability to make plans, and accomplish goals and visions.

Negative fire energy

Power struggles, anger, jealousy, manipulation, aggression and domination disorder the digestion, causing ulcers, diabetes, heat and energy imbalances. Either there is too much transformation, causing destruction, or not enough, causing apathy.

Fire healing

Sun bathing, saunas, sweat lodges, heat treatments, nutrition, diets, moxibustion, stimulating massage, and exercise.

Fire challenge

Rise above power struggles caused by the ego and align to the divine will where consciousness expands to see and feel more than just one's own needs and desires.

Fire elemental emotions

Anger has many faces, from anger, jealousy, rage, competition and aggression, to resentment and blame. These are all associated with positioning and power struggles. The ego is out to get what it wants in its own way and when it wants it. When positive, the fiery emotions warm and lighten the heart so that we can enjoy laughter, joy and creative transformation.

Fire element disease

Excess of the fire element causes liver, gall bladder, pancreas, spleen, and stomach problems, digestive disorders and excess heat. Shortage of the fire element causes an inability to digest food, dampness, cold, lack of energy, absence of passion, and an inability to change.

The Air Element

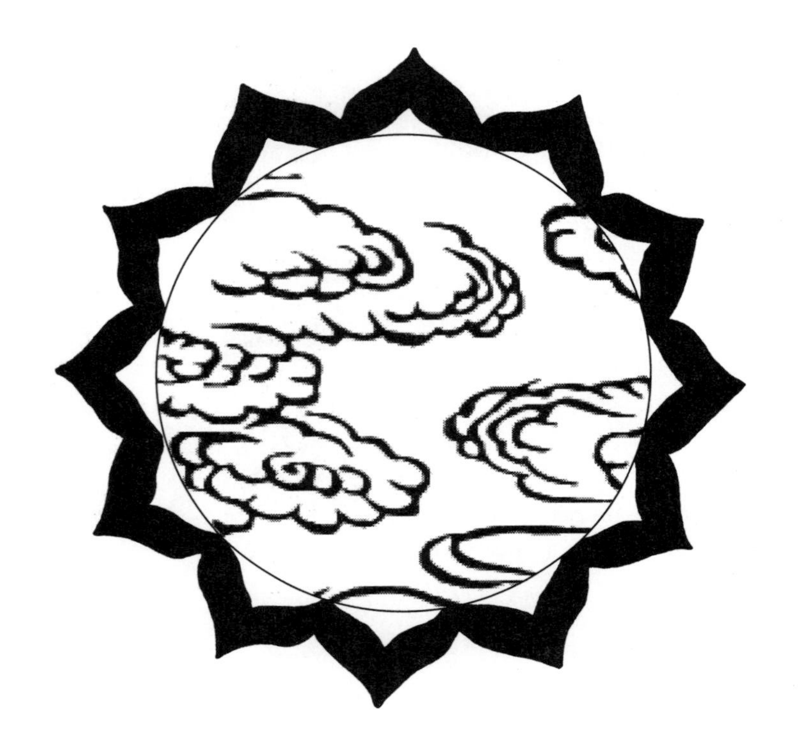

Chakra	Twelve petalled Anahata unstruck chakra
Air body location	Heart, arms, hands
Air dynamic	Yin, feminine, receptive
Air color	Green
Air emotion	Love
Air sense	Touch
Air taste	Sour
Air astrology	Aquarius in the ankles; Libra in the kidneys, ovaries and womb; Gemini in the shoulder, arms and hands

Air energetics

Expansive; dispersing toward equilibrium, calm, and evenness.

Air lessons

We must learn to release the wounds of the heart, forgive and forget so that we can be in the present to give and receive love. When we are in the heart, there is abundance.

Positive air energy

The heart opens, love flows, and giving and receiving abundance becomes a way of life. The air element offers connectedness through respectful relationship, awareness, sensitivity, understanding and unselfishness. It guides us to live, interact and make decisions that consider the needs of others and the planet. It also offers effortless ease which comes from being in the present with faith and trust.

Negative air energy

Greed and speed keep us out of the heart. No matter how fast one moves or how much one accomplishes, there is never enough time, money, love – never enough of anything. The mental and emotional condition is one of starvation, even when there is abundance.

Air healing

Breathing exercises, yoga, oxygen therapy, sea voyages, fresh country, desert, mountain or ocean air, emotional counseling, psychotherapy and bodywork to open the heart, chest, breast and shoulder areas.

Air challenge

The challenge is to give, release emotional wounds, slow down, stay in the present, appreciate what one has, and rejoice in 'being' rather than 'doing.' The insecure, needy, wounded, fearful, angry and helpless child becomes a joyful, playful child of the universe.

Positive air elemental emotions

Compassionate, unconditional love which radiates balance, peace and equilibrium, and considers the needs of others and the planet.

Negative air elemental emotions

Greed hardens the heart, inhibits the ability to give and receive love, and causes selfishness.

Air element disease

Excess of the air element causes speed and greed, breathing disorders, gas in the digestive tract and in the muscles, as well as shoulder, arm and hand problems. Shortage of the air element causes slowness, breathing difficulties and lack of oxygen in the body.

The Ether Element

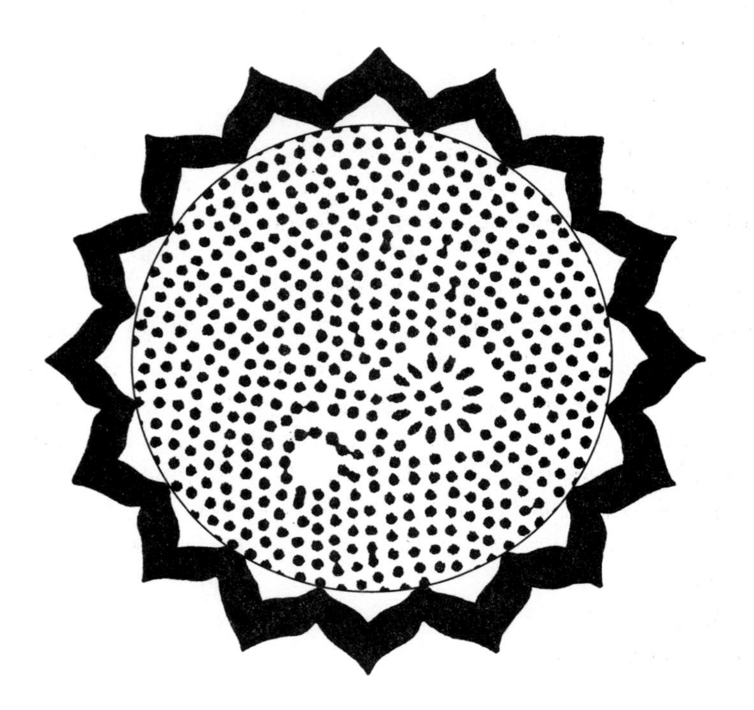

Chakra	Sixteen petalled Vishudda pure chakra
Ether body location	Throat, lungs
Ether dynamic	Yang toward the creation, Yin toward spirituality
Ether color	Turquoise
Ether emotion	Grief toward the creation, longing toward spirituality
Ether sense	Hearing
Ether taste	Bitter
Ether astrology	Elements in balance are directed towards one's highest purpose

Ether energy

This center of purification receives truth from the inner universe, from all the elemental energies, senses and gifts, and from the universe as sound. It then communicates truth with voice, facial expression and subtle energies.

Ether lessons

We can only stand the emptiness of the ether element when we fill it with the invisible qualities of spiritual love and longing; otherwise the emptiness is unbearable and we are forced to fill it with sensual, worldly, emotional and mental activities.

Positive ether energy

Ether is emptiness that receives the wave movements of subtle vibrations of sound, light and warmth. Ether is a state of bliss, balance and truth that is nourished by the gifts of the earthly elements that dissolve into it. Ether longs to dissolve into its source in the spiritual realms. Every aspect of life becomes devoted to achieving this goal and preparing to depart from this world with spiritual awareness. Ether discriminates according to the level of truth it is capable of receiving. Ether also speaks truth, and celebrates spirituality.

Negative ether energy

Indulgent grief, sadness, despair, hopelessness, boredom, and emptiness are fed by fear, attachment, passion and greed.

Ether healing

Sound, music, chanting, beauty, ideals and the invisible energy that is transferred into whatever one does and that permeates one's auric field, clothes, home, possessions and work.

Ether challenge

True spiritual longing makes surrender to the divine will natural and effortless – change is accepted without fear, attachment, anger or greed, and the need for excessive grief is released.

Ether elemental emotions

A sense of loss and temporary grief is a natural feeling, but indulgent grief flows toward the world and becomes entangled in and fed by the negative aspects of earth fear, water attachment, fire anger and air greed.

Ether element disease

Excess ether element causes lung, throat and speaking disorders and emotional imbalances of indulgent grief, boredom, emptiness and longing. Shortage of the ether element causes lack of beauty, grace and care of self, clothes, home and foods, as well as difficulties with speaking and hearing

3

Herbal Instructions

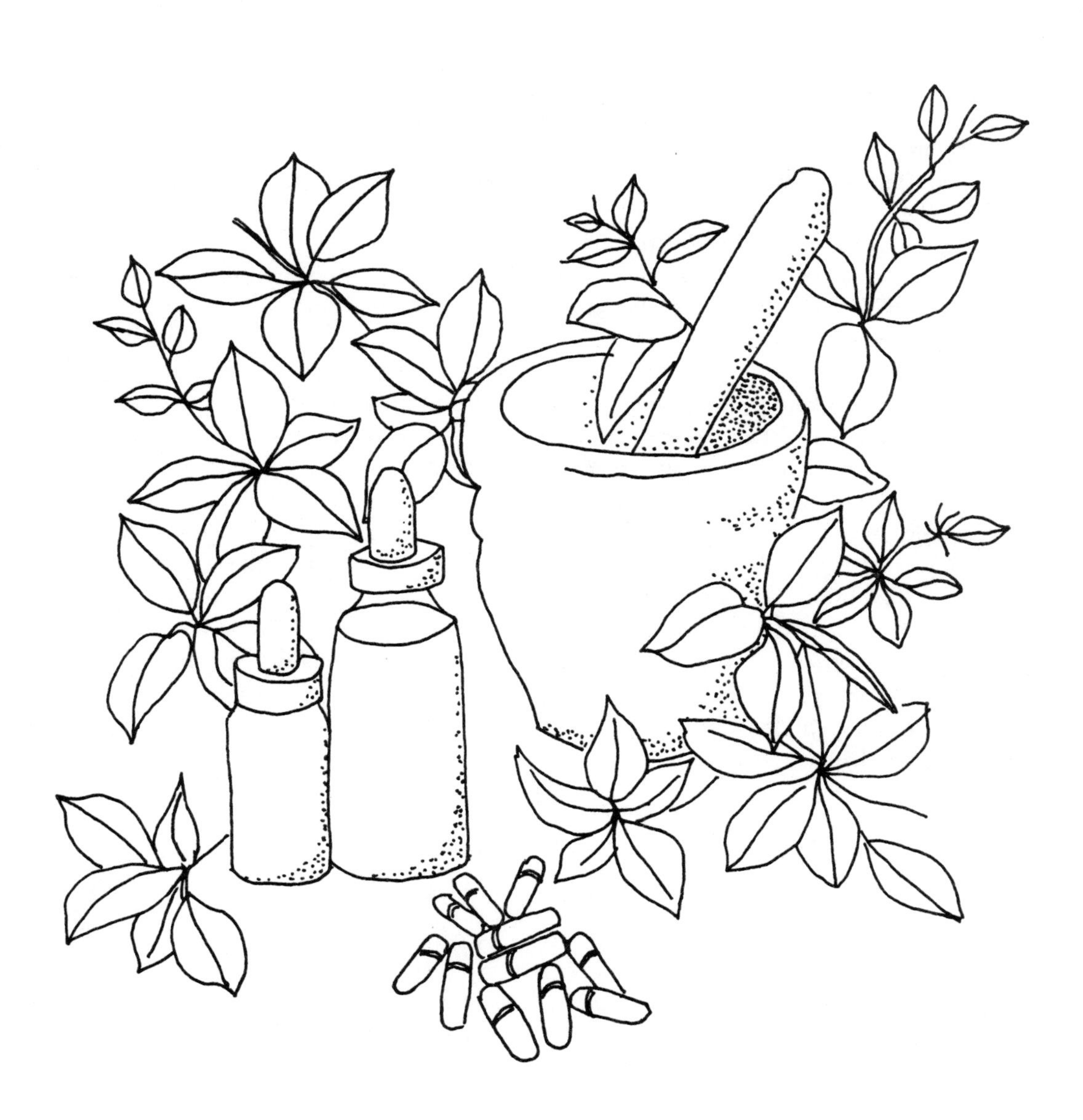

Herbal Instructions

CREATE A RELATIONSHIP WITH HERBS

Before taking herbs it is essential to create a relationship with them. We can welcome them into our life with a ritual or ceremony. We can put them in a special container and visualize their healing energy. It is especially important to accept them as nourishment, so that we can receive them, digest them, and assimilate them for our benefit. We can make them a part of our life in a way that is meaningful to us, read herb books and look at pictures of them, grow them in our gardens, and look for them in the countryside. We can accept plants as our friends and helpers and let them lead us to health and healing.

As we handle the herbs, measure them out, capsule them, make them into pills or take them with our meals, we must treat them with love and respect. The quality of our energy will mix with the herbs. Whenever we look at them, we must look with eyes of love and appreciation, and know that they are '*herbs of grace*' and receive them with gratitude.

The herbal formulae which are given in this book are safe, non–toxic, non–habit–forming herbal nutrients. During the period of transition as we change our diet and begin to take the herbs, however, we must be prepared to monitor our body, be sensitive to changes and needs, and adjust the dosage. If we are under the care of a practitioner, we can communicate any changes or ask for help if we are not sure about something. Using these herbs requires a time of education, transition and guidance, and communication is an important part of that study.

The herbal world is very large. There are thousands of herbs and many different approaches to organizing and using them. We have created a simple, workable system of herbology combined with and supported by nutrition and natural treatments which we present in this book.

As we learn this system we can explore, research and expand its range to include other herbs and treatments we learn from books, teachers and experience. Meanwhile we can read, study and apply this system with confidence as we create a foundation for health.

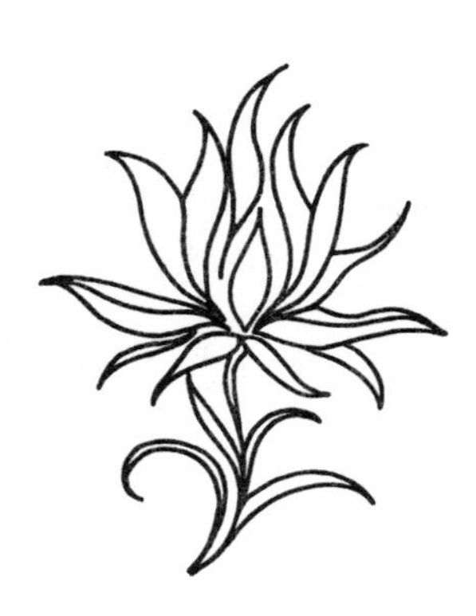

HERBAL POWDERS

In our Herbs of Grace school pharmacy and dispensary we prepare the herbal formulae in powder form from wildcrafted organic herbs in small amounts so that they are fresh. Because we believe they are more effective and potent in their pure state, we do not tincture them or send them to factories to be bound with fillers, to be heated or pressure tableted. We offer fresh, pure, unprocessed herbs from plants growing in their natural habitat.

We encourage you to be your own home herbalist and involve yourself in the preparation of your herbs. You are also welcome to prepare the formulae for your own use by following the proportions given in this book. The time and energy that you contribute to your own healing will be reflected in the results.

If you cannot take powders in liquid or in capsules because of difficulty swallowing or because of a sensitive digestive system, you can swallow them with a Slippery Elm drink, mix the dry herbs with honey, melted butter or Slippery Elm, or make tinctures or extracts from the powders. If you do not wish to capsule them yourself we offer a capsuling service at an extra charge to cover the cost of the capsules and the labor. We believe that if you become involved in your own healing by making your own herbal tablets or capsules, you are increasing the positive healing energy of the herbs. It is important to recognize that time, love and energy focused on the herbs increases their ability to contribute to your health and well–being.

It is also true that you receive greater value for money with fresh herbs because you are not paying for expensive manufacturing processes, packaging, advertising, storage, shipping and sales commissions. We offer products that are pure, fresh and simple. The results speak directly instead of through fancy packaging or advertising that the customer also pays for. We don't need advertising because clients order again and again and recommend the products once they have experienced their value.

If you are going to make up your own formulae, buy fresh, wildcrafted organic herbs and grind them in an electric coffee mill or a Vita Mix. Some herbs are so hard that you will not be able to grind them and you may have to pulverize them in some other way, or purchase them in powdered form. It takes effort and investment to set up your own herbal pharmacy and to research sources for all the herbs required in the formulae. We do not sell individual powders, so you need to make your own contacts with health food stores, herbal growers and wildcrafters if you wish to make your own formulae.

Our School of Natural Medicine home study courses offer training to help you set up your own herbal pharmacy and dispensary. We encourage you to enroll as well as to attend our Summer School in August. Many clients have become students of the School of Natural Medicine and trained to become holistic health practitioners and educators after experiencing the benefits of this system of natural medicine in restoring and maintaining health.

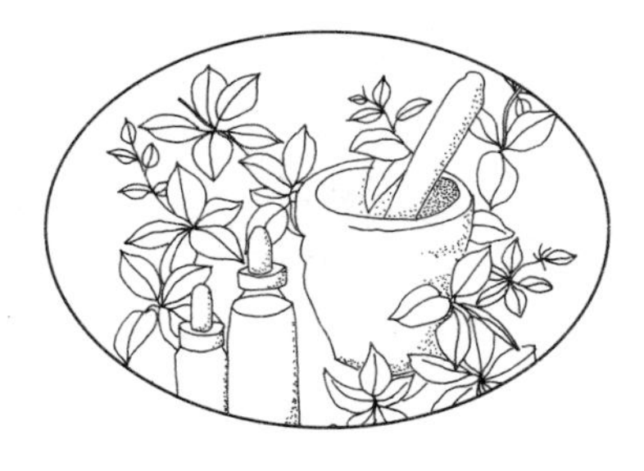

CAPSULING

Capsules are small cylindrical containers into which the powdered herb is compressed. Manufacturers make them in various sizes. We recommend capsule size 0 or 00. Capsules are readily available in drugstore pharmacies and health food stores in non–vegetarian gelatin form. It is also possible to purchase capsules made of a vegetable or seaweed gel in most health food stores. There are two ways of filling capsules which are described below.

Capsuling Method 1:

Put the powders in a dish at least one half to one inch deep, or leave them in the plastic package and fill them from there. Open up the capsule, holding one half in each hand. Press each half of the capsule down into the powder, and tap several times so that the powder is pressed up inside. When both parts of the capsule are as full as possible press the two halves together again to make a finished edible capsule. Do not scoop as this will make the powder fly like dust. If the powder makes you sneeze or affects your mucus membranes, use an inexpensive paper painter's mask, which you can purchase at low cost from a hardware or paint store.

Capsuling Method 2:

Use a capsuling device which you can purchase at a health food store or the Herbs of Grace pharmacy at the School of Natural Medicine.

OTHER METHODS OF POWDER PREPARATION

Honey Tablets

Many herbalists prefer to mix the powders into a ball with honey. Make up the honey pills in daily amounts, because there are no preservatives. Pinch off the dose and roll between the fingers before swallowing. Take the pills immediately before eating.

Butter Tablets

This ancient Indian method of pill making is easy and pleasant. Mix the powder in melted ghee or butter, shape into a roll and refrigerate. Divide into doses per meal, then roll into balls that are smooth and easy to swallow.

Slippery Elm Tablets

Take the daily amount of powder and mix with approximately one–third Slippery Elm, add distilled water, form into a roll of herbal compound and then pinch off into pills to roll between your fingers. Make only enough for each day because there is no preservative in the mixture. Even if herbs mixed with Slippery Elm are stored overnight in a fridge they will spoil.

Drinking Powders

Some patients prefer to take the powders straight, either with juice, water, liquid yogurt or kefir. Mix the powder in just enough liquid to blend, swallow quickly and follow with a chaser.

Others report that a straw works wonders to get the mixture down easily as it bypasses the taste buds and doesn't stick in the mouth.

The bitter taste actually contributes healing benefits because it influences the taste buds on the tongue, causing reflex stimulation to the gastrointestinal tract. Because we have unbalanced tastes due to excessive cravings for sweet, salt or sour, the bitter and pungent tastes help balance the taste buds and our digestive processes. According to Ayurveda philosophy it is essential for good health to have all five tastes available regularly in our diet. After a week this method becomes easier. We recommend it whenever possible, except when capsules or tablets are more convenient for work or travel.

Over the years I have worked with hundreds of clients who prefer powders. I have known people who sprinkle the herbs on their food or put the powders into their mouth and then swallow them with water or another liquid. Many have reported that they love the taste of the herbs and that it makes them feel good. Explore the possibilities and use the system that works best for you. Certainly if you can endure the strong taste for a week or so you will find that you not only get used to it, but that you actually enjoy the flavor.

Herbal Brews

The Chinese method of brewing herbs may also be used if warm herbal tea is preferred. Put the daily dose in a container and pour boiling water over it, then mix and steep. Drink throughout the day. Although there is some change of chemistry due to the heat and the steeping, the results are excellent. The added advantage is the continuous beneficial influence of the tastes on the tongue and on the digestive system.

Experiment and try different methods. Be flexible. At different times it may be preferable to take the powders in different ways.

Dosage

Average Monthly Dose

An average dose for an adult of medium size with reasonable health is about one ounce of herbs per week. This amount can be increased if higher amounts of nutritional or rejuvenative herbs, such as the Multi–Mineral Vitamins Naturally, Stomach Acid Alkaline, Adrenal or Nerve formulae are required. This makes the monthly dose anywhere from four to eight ounces. This can be increased if the person is large or very active or wishes to pursue a dedicated program of purification and regeneration. Several different formulae are mixed together to provide nutrients to balance the inner ecology as determined by an iris analysis. Start off with average amounts and then adjust according to response and need.

Chronic Monthly Dose

Doses for chronic conditions such as arthritis, rheumatism, colitis or nervous exhaustion can be as high as three ounces per week, or as much as the individual can take. This depends on digestive capability, food habits, symptoms, age, pain levels and many other considerations.

How to Work Out the Daily Dose

1. Divide the herbal powders equally into four plastic baggies, one bag for each week of the month.
2. Take one week's bag and divide the powders into seven piles, one for each day.
3. Once you have worked out the daily dose, divide it by two, three or more, depending on how many times you wish to take the herbs with food during the day.
4. Decide how you wish to take the herbs, then prepare them in daily or weekly amounts.
5. Take individual doses immediately before meals, or with the first bite or two of food.
6. Do not swallow the herbs more than two minutes before eating, or at the end of the meal. If you forget and take them after a meal, eat more food after swallowing the herbs.
7. Once you know your daily amount for this series of herbs there is no need to divide any more of the weekly bags. Take the daily dose during the day with food.

Kidney Formulae Dose

Sometimes, it is important that kidney herbs go directly to the kidneys without being processed with food digestion. Take one half teaspoon, or two capsules, with a cup of liquid between meals, two times a day. They can also be included in the herbal nutrient mix.

Bowel Formulae Dose

Take this separately to control the dosage. Individuals respond differently depending on whether they are constipated or have diarrhea. Start with one half teaspoon or two capsules, two or three times a day, and adjust as needed. Strong cases of constipation may require as many as thirty capsules per day until natural peristalsis returns. Diarrhea may need as little as one capsule per day. The average amount for those on a rejuvenation program is about two capsules per meal. Start with the average amount and adjust as needed.

Herbs for Infants and Children

The earlier children experience the taste of herbs the better. If they get used to the bitter and pungent tastes as well as the delicate herbal flavors, they will be receptive to using them for the rest of their lives. I have known many women who have used herbs during their months of pregnancy and breast feeding, in tea and tincture form, with excellent results and no problems. Once children are willing to take herbs on their own, Catnip/Fennel and Wild Lettuce/Valerian herbal tinctures or teas work wonders when there is gas, nervous digestion or sleeplessness.

Sometimes children cannot, or will not swallow tablets or capsules. Tinctures are the best alternative, and the small amounts they need can be dropped in juice. Even easier to take are pleasant herb teas, homeopathic remedies, aromatherapy essences and flower remedies. Children respond directly and quickly to small amounts of these natural remedies.

Over many years of practice I have worked with young children who became very involved in their healing process. During the consultation they enjoyed the questions and the attention, and they loved to see a drawing or a photo of their own iris. Using the self–magnifying mirror, I would show them their own eyes. Then I would take them into the pharmacy and dispensary, and after showing them how we mix the herbs I would ask them how they wanted to take them.

They would know what they were willing to do. Sometimes I would let them try a tincture or a capsule and ask for their cooperation, telling them I would give them the herbs only if they wanted to take them. Almost always they said they would take them and they did. Herbs became a part of their life at a very young age. I asked them to decorate and draw in their copy of *Herbs of Grace* and each week they would show me their art work. Wonderful relationships developed and healing manifested in a loving way which became a pleasant memory for them.

Success depends on how you present the herbs to the children. My experience was that they became very happy and excited about using plants and taking responsibility for their own healing. You cannot push children who are set on resistance, so the best way is to gain their cooperation and make their healing an adventure they enjoy.

Dosage Guidelines for Children

1. *Up to one year:* one drop of tincture in water one to three times a day, or pinches of herb powder mixed together with carob powder and taken in juice or with mashed fruit.

2. *Up to two years:* two drops of tincture in water two to four times a day, or two pinches of powder in juice or with fruit.

3. *From two to seven years:* four drops of tincture in water two to six times a day as needed, half a capsule of powder mixed with carob powder and taken in juice or with fruit, or a capsule of powder twice a day.

4. *From seven to twelve years:* six to eight drops of tincture in water one to eight times a day, or a capsule of powder four times a day.

5. *From twelve onward:* it is possible to take a minimum adult dose of about twelve drops of tincture in water three times a day, or two capsules three times a day with food. However, always consider the individual, their size, the condition of their digestive system, the state of their health and their present health or illness. Try smaller doses and adjust to larger amounts. Use common sense as well as written instructions.

Herbs for the Elderly, Chronically Ill or the Dying

When the elderly, the dying and those with chronic conditions are involved, nourishment and treatment must be adjusted sensitively. Doses, as with children, are reduced. Start out with one half the normal adult dose of herbs, and adjust according to response and need.

Treatment for those who are dying must be monitored and supported with wisdom and genuine caring. While the time for healing and cure may be over, much can be done to ease them during the preparation and passing. The essential work is to keep the eliminative channels flowing, support the liver and ease any pain crises. Basic treatment suggestions are as follows:

1. Digestion may be sensitive and herbs may need to be taken with Slippery Elm drinks.

2. Therapeutic herbal and aromatherapy baths together with reflexology and massage will help keep circulation and lymph moving when those you are caring for are bedridden or unable to exercise

3. Lobelia baths and poultices reduce pain.

4. Coffee enemas reduce many symptoms by activating the bowels and liver.

5. Flower essences and homeopathy ease fear, anxiety and tension and help patients to surrender to their departure from this world and welcome their entrance into spirit.

6. Purifying and mono diets, and fresh juices, are easy to digest and nutritious.

The simple diets and treatments given in this book will help relatives and friends to care for their loved ones who are in deep life/death transition.

Above all, when you are caring for the dying, remember that it is the love and respect for their process that will speak directly to their heart and soul. Surround them with love and touch. Make their room beautiful. Bring color, fresh air and fragrance to their last days. Read to them. Play uplifting music. Pray together. Talk to them from your heart. Tell them all that you always wanted to tell them. Reminisce. Inspire them to release their physical body and embrace the life of the spirit. Tell them you love them. Let them go. Do not try to hold them back. Tell them that you will be fine after they leave and that they don't need to worry. Put soft fragrant candles and flowers in their room and open the windows to the sun and the stars. As they slip away from this world, let their last experiences be of gentleness, sweetness and love.

HERBAL DECOCTIONS

Decoctions are strong herbal brews that bring out the virtues from whole or cut roots, barks and berries. When they are powdered they can be infused or simmered gently for a short time and then left to steep. Decoctions are used for drinks, baths, enemas, poultices and fomentations.

If you wish to make a decoction of cut or whole berries, roots or barks and the plant material is not powdered, simmer the herb very, very gently over a very low flame so that the virtue of the herb or herbs will be released without destroying the potency or value. Use only glass or stainless steel containers. Small seeds like Fenugreek need about twenty minutes, and roots which are very hard may take about thirty to forty–five minutes.

Decoction proportions are approximately thirty grams, or one ounce of herb, per one pint of water, or one–half ounce per cup. Start out with two pints so that one pint will boil off during the simmering.

HERBAL TEAS, TISANES OR INFUSIONS

Herbal teas are used for many purposes; delightful drinks, enemas, baths, poultices, and as medicinal support during acute crises or chronic conditions. They can be made from powders, leaves, roots and barks or even from tinctures or aromatherapy oils. They can be individual herbs, mixtures of two or more herbs, or formulae made up of numerous herbs. The best approach

is to start simple, try a few herbs, get to know them, and then expand the repertoire. It is best to try recipes and commercial blends until we find our way and learn to enjoy the creative art of natural herbal beverage blending.

Proportions vary according to taste and depend upon the part of the plant used, its purpose, freshness and potency. The general rule is to use one teaspoon of herb per cup of tea. Many prefer half that amount of herb for enjoyment and double that when there is a medicinal need. If you are using the herbal teas for enemas, poultices, baths or fomentations, use a higher dose of herbs per cup of liquid, from one to two teaspoons per cup of liquid.

Pour boiling water over the herbs. Use a glass or stainless steel tea pot so that chemical reactions will not take place within the container. Porous metals such as aluminum are unsuitable for use with herbs. Steep longer than for ordinary tea, at least twelve minutes. Pour off the beverage through a strainer. Glass tea pots make elegant containers that show off the beauty and color of the herbs. Add flowers like hibiscus, chrysanthemum, violets or rose petals for beauty and fragrant taste.

Leave the herbs in the container and add fresh amounts of boiling water, then add more herbs as required during the day. Clean out the pot at the end of the day and start fresh the next morning. Honey or maple syrup is pleasant. Add grape or apple juice to the herbal beverage to make it more satisfying and strengthening, especially in cold or damp weather. If you are using barks or roots and they are not ground into a powder, make a decoction, strain and add into the tea. Don't mix them during the preparation.

If you are having a party and want to serve a delightful herbal juice punch, try my favorite recipe: apple juice, red grape juice, orange and lemon juice mixed with Hibiscus, Lemon Grass, Peppermint, Ginger and Rose Hips. Add a dash of Cinnamon and Allspice. Float a few orange and lemon rings, mull to a moderate, warm temperature, or serve iced. Your guests will appreciate this delicious and satisfying drink.

Herbal Tea Formulae

DIGESTEA – This delightful tea improves the digestive chemistry, balances the acid/alkaline secretions in the stomach, improves digestion and increases the assimilation of nutrients. Take a cup one quarter hour before, or half an hour after, eating or anytime throughout the day.

Meadowsweet, Wood Betony, Peppermint, Hibiscus, Lemon Grass, Rose Hips and Fennel

SERENITEA – If you would like to relax before sleep, try one or two cups of this tea before retiring. Because it is a strong but pleasant tasting tea, milk and honey improves the flavor. This is a useful tea to have on hand to weather stress, crises or emotional upsets.

Catnip, Vervain, Mistletoe, Peppermint, Wood Betony (3), Valerian (0.5), Scullcap (0.5) and Hops (0.5)

WATERBALANCE – This mildly diuretic tea beneficially influences the entire urinary tract and helps regulate the elimination of water. Acute cystitis can be helped by drinking a cup every half an hour until the symptoms are relieved.

Couchgrass, Parsley Leaves, Clivers, Buchu, Uva Ursi and Chickweed

Individual Herbal Teas

Chickweed – Neutralizes and eliminates acidity.

Ginger – Fresh Ginger increases body heat and improves digestion.

Licorice – A gentle aperient for children and adults that also stabilizes blood sugar; take six cups a day for hypoglycemic conditions.

Mullein – Slows diarrhea and balances bowel function.

Oat Straw – A high source of silica and calcium, add it to teas and use in water cure full baths and footbaths.

Red Clover – An excellent blood purifier that combines well with Red Raspberry during purification programs.

Red Raspberry – The high iron content attracts oxygen and increases metabolic activity, overcoming sluggishness; excellent for pregnant women; add to teas during pregnancy and for strength during and after menstrual periods.

Rose Hips – Add to tea blends to provide vitamin C during colds and infections.

Sage – This ancient Chinese longevity tea stimulates cerebral circulation and increases brain activity and memory.

Oils and Ointments

Balm of Gilead Ointment – Soothes and heals eczema, psoriasis, sores, cracked skin and open wounds.

Chickweed Ointment – Relieves heat, itching and rashes.

Comfrey Ointment – Aids cell growth, and the repair of cuts, wounds and fractures; provides regenerative nutrients directly where it is needed.

Garlic Oil – Useful for warts, pimples and infected wounds; apply directly on areas two to three times per day; combine with Mullein oil for ear infections.

Mullein Oil – Two to three drops in the ear relieve earache, suppuration and inflammation of the ear, especially when combined with Garlic oil. It can also be applied externally on sprains, bruises, sores, swollen glands, aching joints and skin diseases.

Baths, Footbaths and Hand Baths

The use of herbs in these naturopathic water cure treatments is covered in the Herbal and Naturopathy Treatment chapter along with the recommended herbs. During my studies and purifications at *Rainbow Island* and *Healing Waters* healing centers, we bathed regularly in Chaparral herbal baths, absorbing the purifying herb directly through our skin. Lobelia baths produce deep relaxation during crises, trauma or exhaustion. Chickweed baths relieve itching and skin discomfort. Hand and foot baths draw the nutrients immediately into the capilliary circulation and then quickly into the blood stream. Make herbal baths an important part of home therapeutics.

Herbal Formulae Tinctures

ANTISPASMODIC – Useful for shocks, cramps, spasms, hysteria, asthma and heart attacks.

Lobelia, Scullcap, Black Cohosh, Cayenne, Gum Myrrh, Catnip and Cramp Bark

DIGESTIVE – Relieves colic, wind and discomfort in the stomach. Excellent for children.

Catnip and Fennel

NERVINE NUTRIENT – Feeds and calms the nervous system and reduces hyperactivity. Rub on the back of the neck to influence the medulla regulatory center and calm breathing and basic body functions.

Black Cohosh, Lady's Slipper, Scullcap, Lobelia and Blue Vervain

NERVINE RELAXANT – Calms the nervous system when sleep or digestion are disturbed.

Wild Lettuce and Valerian

Individual Herbal Tinctures

Echinacea – Assists the lymphatic defense system during acute infections, colds, flu.

Euphrasia – An excellent eye wash to brighten and strengthen the eyes.

Elder flower – The highest herbal source of potassium, Elderflower complements treatment for excess acidity, fibroids and nutritional imbalance; helps to maintain a youthful and supple skin.

Lobelia – By prescription only, for use as an internal emetic when combined with Peppermint tea (do not attempt an emetic without professional advice), and to relieve asthma by rubbing over congested areas to relieve pain, spasms and swelling; use as a poultice over the lung area to relieve congestion, inflammation, pain and coughing.

Myrrh – Rub into gums after brushing the teeth or use a dropper in dental cleaning equipment solutions; good for bleeding gums, pyorrhea, sores, pimples and herpes.

Saw Palmetto – A specific for the mammary glands, it complements treatment for breast lumps and swollen breasts. Take internally and rub on the breasts.

Wild Yam – Relieves digestive flatulence, bloating, colic and cramps; high in progesterone; useful to relieve hot flashes, prevent osteoporosis and balance hormones during menopause.

Tincture Dosage

Drop the tincture dose in a glass and pour boiling water over it. Steep at least five minutes so that the alcohol can be evaporated before drinking. Swish it around in the mouth, allowing the taste buds to benefit from the flavor as it is mixed with saliva, then swallow. Tinctures are administered according to age, three to four times per day as required or more often in acute conditions. Size, weight and sensitivity are also considerations.

Up to two years of age:

Two drops in water, one to two times per day.

From two years to seven years of age:

Four drops in water, one to three times per day.

Between seven years and twelve years of age:

Use six to eight drops in water, one to four times per day.

The full adult dose is:

Use six, twelve or eighteen drops in water, three, six or nine times daily as required.

Acute Conditions:

Dosage can be increased to every five, ten or fifteen minutes minutes, half hour, hour, and so on, depending on the need, symptoms and response. Seek professional guidance.

4

Herbal Ecology

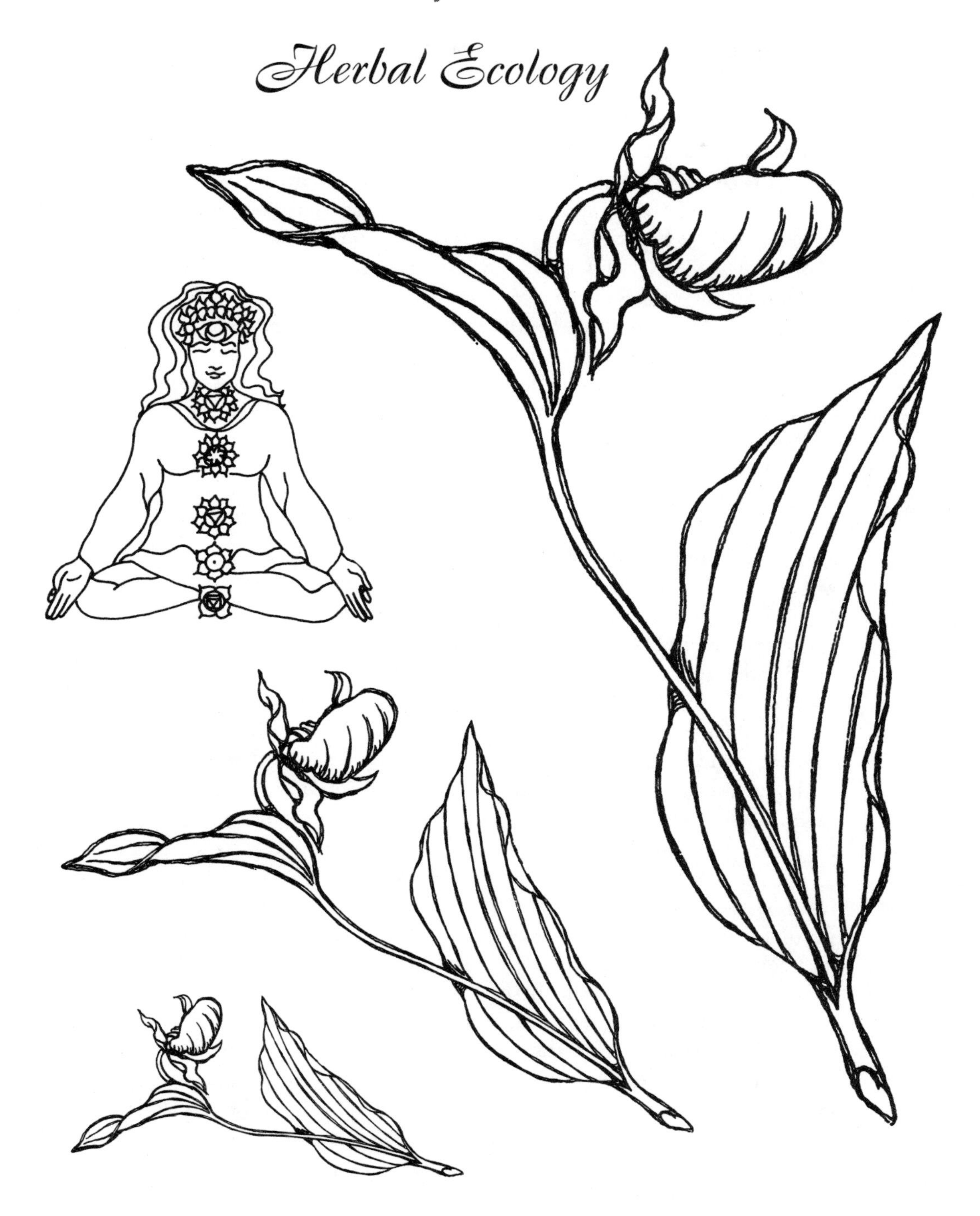

Herbal Ecology

This chapter introduces the herbal formulae I created as well as the individual herbs I most often recommend when appropriate. The formulae, both individually and in combination, have all been tried and tested for many years, first by myself and students and graduates of the School of Natural Medicine, and then with thousands of patients all over the world. The results of all the formulae have been consistently positive, safe and effective. They are offered for the benefit of humanity. Their positive healing action harmonizes the inner ecology of each individual, so that they can make a contribution of balance, peace and health to the world ecology.

The herbal formulae are nutritional, non–toxic and non–habit–forming. They are a highly superior and specific form of natural nutrition to be taken either during a course of purification and rejuvenation or as regular food supplements.

The herbal formulae are amphoteric, which means they are balancing. Whether underactive or overactive, individual organs, body systems and glands are restored to normal function by the use of specific and appropriate formulae that contain a supportive blend of activation, elimination and nutritional rejuvenation. The body takes what it needs, when and where it needs it, from the nutrients offered by the formulae.

The key to the use of these formulae is the vision of the inner ecology as given through the study and practice of iridology. Through the eyes, the holographic window of body, emotions, mind and soul, we are given a glimpse of our inner world, the constitutional fabric of life, and the function of our glands, organs and systems.

When we use herbal formulae guided by this knowledge–wisdom–vision, it is important that we blend an individual mix that contains all the nutrients necessary to balance the inner ecology. Through our understanding of the constitutional types, the eliminative organs and other organs, systems and glands, we blend a mix that contains herbs to stimulate and support the process of purification, regeneration and transformation.

First, the constitutional type tells us the basic formulae which are required to compensate for inherent weaknesses. Next, the iris clearly shows which organs, systems and glands are in need of balancing herbal formulae to activate, purify, rebuild and rejuvenate. Other iris markings and colors guide the practitioner to add other formulae to the nutrient mix so that the entire inner ecology is nourished. The best results are obtained when the body is receiving all that it needs to enable it to return to balanced and harmonious function.

Whenever iridologists trained by the School of Natural Medicine analyze clients' eyes, they first determine the constitutional type or types. They then determine which eliminative channels are overfunctioning or underfunctioning. Herbs are blended to strengthen the constitution and restore balanced elimination. They also take care to include other formulae or individual herbs if any other major organs, glands or systems reveal weakness or unbalanced function, or if the client has strong symptoms. Further iridology information can be found in the Iridology chapter.

While it is best to take the herbs under the guidance of a qualified Natural Physician/ Naturopath/Iridologist/Herbalist, if you decide to do–it–yourself by taking individual or combined formulae based on your symptoms, or intuition, please take into consideration the dosage and preparation instructions presented in the Herbal Instruction chapter. With careful and conscious monitoring of responses you will be able to determine which herbs will be helpful to you.

Formulae Proportions

It is my belief that herbs belong to everyone and that formulae should not be kept secret. We offer the exact formulae proportions and invite you to make up formulae for your own use. You are also welcome to order retail and blend your own nutrient combinations, or come for a consultation and receive your individual nutrient mix as a part of a natural medicine health prevention and rejuvenation program.

All herbs are combined in equal parts except where otherwise stated in parentheses, i.e. (0.5) means half a part. The sample formula below means: 6 parts Horsetail, 4 parts Oatstraw, 3 parts Comfrey, 1 part Lobelia, 2 parts Marshmallow root, 1 part Kelp, 1 part Parsley root.

Horsetail (6), Oatstraw (4), Comfrey (3), Lobelia, Marshmallow root (2), Kelp and Parsley root

Practitioner Information

Because trained practitioners combine the herbs into personal nutrient mixes, using from five to nine formulae together to balance the inner ecology, the repeated use of stimulating hot herbs has been limited or deleted from many of the formulae. If a formulae is used individually and does not contain stimulating herbs such as Cayenne, Garlic or Ginger, these may be added whenever they are needed.

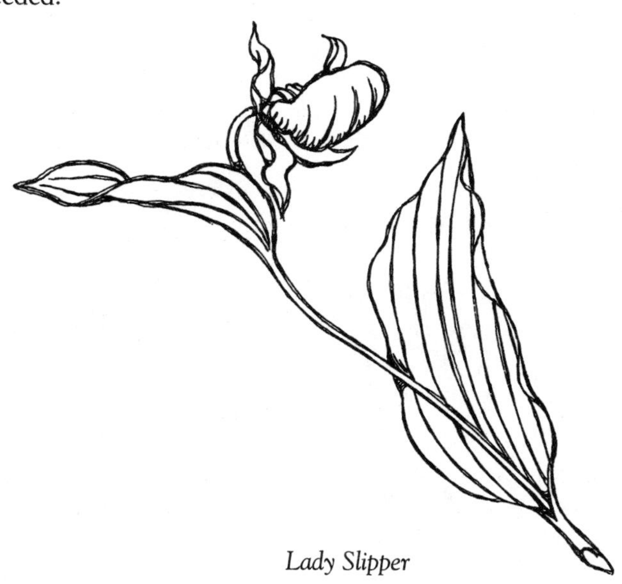

Lady Slipper

Allergy Cautions

It is important to determine whether you have sensitivity to stimulating hot spices or foods, allergies, liverish reactions after eating fried foods, oils or fats, or whether you have excess liver heat as defined by Chinese medicine. If you have this sensitivity make up the formulae without any of the strong hot herbs such as Cayenne, Ginger, Cloves, Garlic, and Ginseng. You can also test yourself or your client with a pendulum or kineseology.

Digestive Cautions

Whenever there is extreme digestive sensitivity it is wise to administer the herbs with a warm drink made from one teaspoon of Slippery Elm mixed with one cup of warm water, or soy, rice or almond milk, and honey. This soothes their passage through the stomach and intestines until the healing of the gastrointestinal tract has strengthened the system.

Take the herbs immediately before eating so that the saliva and digestive juices mix the herbs with the food. If you forget and take them after your meal, we recommend eating more food right after taking the herbs. If you do not have a full meal three times a day, take the herbs with a healthy snack. You can also take them more often. As long as the daily dose of herbs is taken throughout the day, suit yourself as to how often or when. Do not take them on an empty stomach until your system is used to them. Eventually most people can take them with water or juice, or even when on a fast. Best results are achieved when herbs are combined with restorative changes in diet and living habits.

Adrenal Formula

In these days of stress, nervous tension, anxiety and hyperactivity, the adrenal glands take a beating whenever we run on our nerves. This formula provides the nutrients to strengthen, support and rebuild the adrenal glands, which deal with stress and stimulate the response required to deal with the situation. Whenever you are in conflict, face deadlines, emergencies, trauma, or long–term survival flight–or–fight stress, this formulae will support the adrenals. This is also a nourishing, balancing formula to restore normal function to either hypoactive adrenals contributing to systemic exhaustion, or hyperactive adrenals at the mercy of a sympathetic dominant nervous system, in continuous sensitive response to stressful outside stimuli.

Adrenal and nerve herbs help clients to become increasingly aware of their depletion and exhaustion, especially if the use of stimulants that flog the adrenals into forced activity are discontinued. Support healing transition during this time by resting and avoiding unnecessary activities. Do not push the river; learn to flow with it.

Borage, Mullein, Lobelia, Ginseng, Gotu Kola, Hawthorn berries and Parsley root

Alkaline Formula

"From the ocean cometh all life," Dr. Shook says in his *Treatise on Herbology*, inspiring respect for the nutritional value of seaweeds, which contain almost the full range of basic nutrients that are required by the human body. From this range of nutrients the body selects what it needs. A valuable source of trace elements, this formula is effective whenever the iris or symptoms indicate an imbalance of chemistry, or a lack of some essential mineral or trace element. This formula will help to balance acid/alkaline, normalize body chemistry, relieve arthritis and rheumatism, and improve nutritional imbalances. It is also useful as an additive in herbal tablet making or poultices because its hygroscopic properties help to form a cohesive mixture.

Irish Moss, Kelp, Iceland Moss and Bladderwrack

Allergy Formula

Whenever the immune system is overburdened the body reacts to aggravating stimuli with acute reactions such as hay fever, rashes or uncomfortable mucus discharges. Although it is essential to adjust diet and living habits, the force of the discomfort can be alleviated with this formula. There is no substitute for treating the cause of the distress, so unless the body system is cleared and returned to balanced function a true cure cannot take place. For best results use this formula for foundation level treatment in combination with other formulae for restoration of active normal function of the eliminative channels and regeneration of any weak or unbalanced body glands, systems and organs.

Black Pepper, Burdock root, Cinnamon, Elecampagne, Ephaedra, Ginger root, Licorice root and Marshmallow root

Anemia Formula

This formula provides strength and power to a sluggish system and helps to restore an adequate supply of iron necessary for body metabolism and energy. Especially valuable to pregnant and nursing mothers, this formula provides assimilable iron that does not cause side effects such as constipation. The formula contains all the additional ingredients to utilize the iron in the system. Avoid caffeine in any form when you are iron deficient because it leaches iron from your body. Also avoid it when you are taking iron herbs because it neutralizes the buildup of increased iron.

Barberry, Comfrey root, Sarsaparilla, Sassafras, Cayenne, Quassia root, Yellow Dock root and Lobelia (0.5)

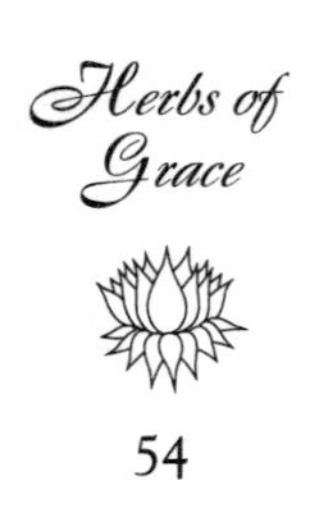

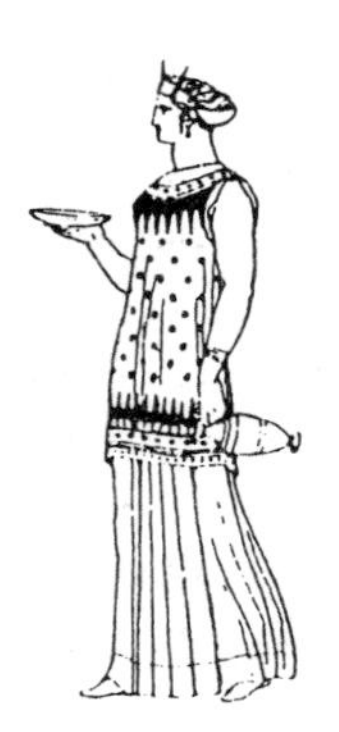

Antibiotics Naturally Formula

Whenever acute distress requires strong activation of the lymphatic immune defense system, this formula provides an alternative to synthetic antibiotics, if used in combination with naturopathic first aid techniques and an understanding of the body cleansing required to relieve obstructions to faulty elimination. It is essential that the bowels are cleansed with enemas and stomach juices are neutralized and purified with Peppermint and Thyme tea. Hot Mustard baths that are followed by steaming under quilts will produce a copious skin elimination which will relieve a burdened system. Other complementary treatments are recommended depending on whether there is fever, sore throat, pain, cough, nausea, inflammation or swelling. It is also important to consult your practitioner.

This formula cannot work effectively when there are toxic accumulations, but if the elimination is activated, and the patient is cleansing with herb teas, lemon water and/or fresh juice, there is an excellent chance of overcoming symptoms in a natural way.

Tablet, capsule and tincture dosage can be increased in both amount and frequency during an acute crisis. When dental surgery pierced through the root of my tooth and caused a severe infection, I took doses of twenty–four capsules every half hour, about one hundred fifty capsules per day, for a period of four days. My dentist was amazed when the infection was completely cleared up without an abscess. I received the additional benefit of a complete inner–cleanse, so instead of being depleted by an acute illness, I was rejuvenated and restored. These are the benefits of living with nature's natural pharmacy. Every health problem becomes a learning challenge which leaves one with greater understanding to apply in any future situation.

This formula can effectively be combined with my Sore Throat Syrup: simmer hot water, honey, apple cider vinegar, lemon juice, Garlic, Ginger and Cayenne pepper. Gargle thoroughly and then drink. Adjust the proportions according to taste preferences. This combination neutralizes the strong flavors, resulting in a delicious, soothing and healing drink which helps restore the mucous membranes to normal function as well as easing soreness.

Cinnamon, Sassafras, Sarsaparilla, Cloves, Mullein, Licorice root, Aniseed, Fennel and Peppermint may also be added to suit individual tastes and needs. Also eat Garlic fresh, sauteed or in soups in high doses during the acute condition. This will effectively reduce infection in the gastrointestinal tract, and help the formula to do its work within the entire body system.

Golden Seal root, Burdock root, Lobelia, Mullein, Poke root, Chaparral, Cayenne, Echinacea root(2) and Thyme (0.5)

Anti-inflammatory Formula

Inflammation is the result of congestion of fluids, irritation, injury, infection and abnormal changes in body chemistry. It is most often painful. This formula was designed to support constitutional treatment. It also complements the use of the Arthritis and Alkaline formulae as well as formulae individually prescribed to clear the eliminative systems and provide systemic balancing to reduce and heal arthritis and rheumatism.

Containing White Willow bark, the original source of aspirin, the formula reduces inflammation and pain without providing the side effects of stronger synthetic drugs. While the process may take longer and must also be coordinated with diet reform and positive changes in living habits, the results are longer lasting. This formula works best when combined with equal parts of Devil's Claw herb.

White Willow bark, Prickly Ash, Yarrow, Poke root, Elder flowers, Black Cohosh, Nettles, Sarsaparilla and Guiacum

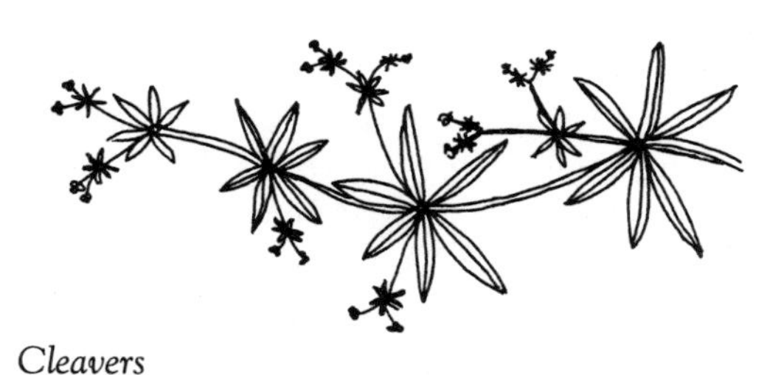

Cleavers

Anti-Weight and Water Formula

This powerful herbal combination seeks to reduce adipose tissue and eliminate excess water without depleting the system. Once the foundation level of treatment has been achieved and the eliminative channels are working efficiently, this formula will support the restoration to normal body weight by increasing the activity of essential body systems that have become sluggish or overburdened. Once weight and water balance are achieved they can be maintained because of the restoration of normal body function.

Problems such as constant eating, anorexia, bulimia, and mentally and emotionally based cravings and addictions must also be addressed through therapy, counseling and flower essences.

Deep and thorough rejuvenation of the gastrointestinal tract will relieve the physical abnormal and constant hunger caused by non–absorption of nutrients through colon walls which are blocked by impacted faeces. Fatigue and exhaustion also contribute to poor eating habits that cause excess weight and water. Systemic constitutional treatment relieves these conditions by establishing normal function. This formula must be supported by other internal herbal formulae, dietary reform, changes in living habits – the complete holistic health program.

Burdock root, Bladderwrack (3), Fennel seeds, Echinacea root, Parsley root and Spirulina

Arthritis Formula

As a complement to systemic treatment, cleansing and diet reform, this formula relieves the discomfort of arthritis and rheumatism. Working to purify the blood, lymph and tissues and reduce inflammation, it helps the system to recover equilibrium of function. The Anti–Inflammatory formula complements the effect of the Arthritis formula.

This formula can also be used as a tea three times a day, or half a cup of the infusion hourly. When discomfort is acute the dosage of capsules may be doubled or tripled.

Oregon Grape root(2), Parsley root, Sassafras, Prickly Ash bark, Black Cohosh root and Ginger root

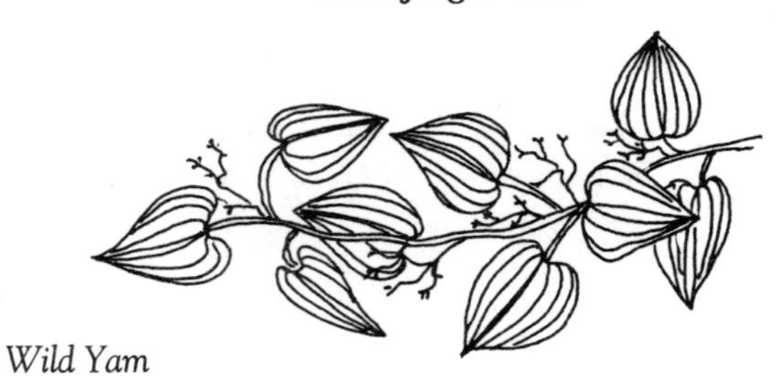

Wild Yam

Asthma Formula

The treatment of asthma is a challenge to the most qualified and experienced practitioner because it involves cleansing, balancing and activation of the eliminative functions, sensitive counseling for mental and emotional causes, and the introduction of living and dietary habits to lessen mucous formation and support the herbal formulae. Treatment for this chronic condition requires the full commitment of the client over about six months. The addition of this formula to systemic treatment steps up the success rate as it encourages the thinning, loosening and expelling of excess mucus from the lungs.

This formula can be taken as a tea (four cups or more per day) depending on need, or in combination with other herbs in capsules or tablets.

It is also useful when used in combination with the Respiratory and Alkaline formulae. Add the Antibiotics Naturally formula if there is evidence of infection, and stop the intake of all mucus forming foods, including sugar, white flour, dairy, coffee, tea and refined, processed foods.

Slippery Elm, Comfrey root, Marshmallow root, Licorice root and Elecampagne (2)

Blood Purifier Formula

Blood purifying herbs help to relieve the blood stream from morbid accumulations which have settled there because of poor dietary and living habits, impaired liver function, and insufficient function of the other eliminative channels, the lymph, bowels, skin and respiratory systems. Whenever the eliminative channels are not functioning properly, toxins accumulate in the blood and tissues and create the climate for infection and disease.

Echinacea root, Oregon Grape root, Poke root, Red Clover blossoms, Sarsaparilla, Sassafras and Yellow Dock root

Body Building Formula

Wherever superior nutrition is needed to provide the raw materials to rebuild damaged or weak bones, muscles and tissue, this formula will provide the means for regeneration. Take internally and apply as poultices directly on affected areas (wounds, damaged vertebrae, broken bones and sprains). If a damaged area does not need to draw nutrients through the blood and lymph, causing congestion, swelling and inflammation, the healing proceeds much more quickly. Because the poultice nutrients are drawn through the skin into the tissues, lymph and circulation of the damaged area, providing nutrients for healing without depleting any other body area or causing excess fluids to be drawn to the damaged areas, inflammation, swelling and pain are reduced and healing progresses more quickly.

Comfrey root, Comfrey leaves, Irish Moss, Marshmallow root, Mullein, Plantain and White Oak bark

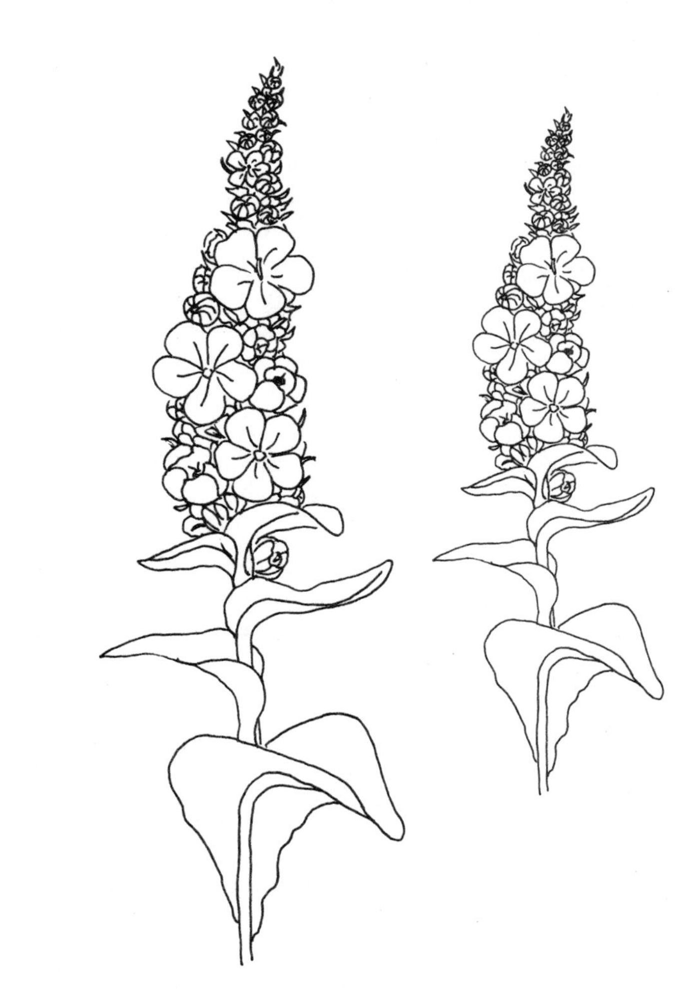

Mullein

Bowel Rejuvenator Formula

Bowel cleansing and rejuvenation are required by almost every human being on a regular basis. The cleaner the colon, the purer the blood stream and lymph, because the walls of the colon allow the absorption of nutrients into the blood and lymph to be distributed throughout the body. A clean colon gives an uplift physically, mentally and emotionally. One feels lighter, cleaner and clearer, and the brain functions better.

This formula normalizes bowel function, whether the problem is constipation or diarrhea which is an indication of more advanced constipation. A colon that is coated with toxic mucus lining is not able to draw off the fluid containing the nutrients, so the feces become more liquid. When the walls of the colon are clean the liquid can be absorbed in a normal way. If diarrhea is persistent use Mullein tea, high doses of Cinnamon sprinkled on applesauce, or baked potatoes. Symptoms often find their source in the colon, and many chronic diseases owe their early development to the accumulation of bowel toxins. If the causes of ill health are cleared, the way to healing opens. Nutrients become available to the body, and the blood and lymph become cleaner. The burden on the eliminative channels becomes less and one's whole being rejoices. "Cleanliness is next to godliness," the old saying goes.

The aim of this formula is to restore normal bowel function, not to create dependence like most laxatives. Because its ingredients work simultaneously to normalize bowel function, tone colon muscles, restore peristalsis, clean bowel pockets and diverticuli, heal raw or inflamed areas and relax areas of tension, it is an overall formula which will ultimately leave the patient without the need to continue the formula. In some cases bowel cleansing may extend to nine months, but often the colon is cleansed, and normal bowel function is restored, in approximately six months. The iris analysis provides an excellent monitoring of this cleansing process.

The bowels should eliminate three movements a day to ensure that fecal matter is not retained in the bowel for more than twelve hours, and that fermentation and absorption of fecal toxins is minimal.

Because this formula accomplishes a very individual result the dosage must be monitored and adjusted according to response and daily changes. In chronic cases of constipation individuals have taken up to 45 capsules per day up to three weeks before their body releases its accumulated fecal matter. This initial release can be aided by the use of the Castor oil pack together with the discriminate use of enemas or colonics.

Caution: Because of its astringent properties Golden Seal should be avoided during pregnancy and nursing, and during regular use should be discontinued after about six weeks. Make the formula without the Golden Seal, add Thyme instead, or use a different bowel formula.

Cascara Sagrada, Ginger root, Golden Seal (or Thyme), Slippery Elm, Turkey Rhubarb, Wahoo (0.25) and Culver's root (0.25)

BOWEL VITALIZER FORMULA

This herbal combination was developed out of a need for a formula which would work as well as Bowel Rejuvenator but not rely on the continued use of Golden Seal, which should not be taken over long periods of time due to its astringent qualities. This formula stimulates bowel elimination through increased liver function. This well–tested formula combines the positive aspects of the Bowel Rejuvenator with a more gentle, less hot, selection of herbs to stimulate natural peristalsis. Adjust dosage according to response. Try out both formulae to see which one suits you better, or alternate the Bowel Rejuvenator with the Bowel Vitalizer.

Caution: During pregnancy make up the formulae without the Mandrake root.

Mandrake root, Ginger root, Licorice root, Wild Yam root and Alfalfa

BURDOCK

Burdock is a specific herb which is given whenever boils, psoriasis, eczema, itch and other skin diseases present strong symptoms. Its strongly purifying influence also increases urine flow, stimulates the lymphatic system and reduces fatty tissue. Use it together with herbs for the kidneys, liver and bowels to purify the blood.

CALAMUS

This herb is added to nutrient mixes whenever flatulence, hyperacidity, fermentation, dyspepsia or bloating present strong symptoms. It is very useful for digestive nervous weakness and works efficiently when combined in equal proportions with Gotu Kola.

CALCIUM FORMULA

A superior intake of calcium is valuable for many conditions including pregnancy, nursing, muscular cramps, hair and nail weakness, and imbalances of body chemistry which lead to weak bones, osteoporosis and calcification of the joints. It is also helpful when babies are teething, because irritability and discomfort are relieved when their bodies have enough calcium to form their teeth without drawing calcium from other areas of their body, causing congestion, pressure on nerves and pain.

Horsetail (6), Oatstraw (4), Lobelia, Marshmallow root (2), Kelp and Parsley root

Cayenne Pepper or Capsicum

This stimulant, antiseptic herb has many valuable uses. As a dietary supplement it increases the circulatory power and provides the means to reach sluggish areas. It is also an essential part of any home herbal first aid kit because of its ability to stem the flow of bleeding or hemorrhage. Heart attacks are relieved by high doses of Cayenne because it equalizes the circulation and increases blood flow.

It is worthwhile to learn about the many uses of this excellent herb that is an essential part of many herbal formulae. *Back to Eden* by Jethro Kloss contains a number of pages devoted to its use. Dr. Raymond Christopher found Cayenne so effective that he wrote a book titled *Capsicum*. However, it is important not to overdo the use of Cayenne in formulae or when taken on its own. Extreme use of any herb, however beneficial, will create imbalances and cause reactions.

Caution: Take care when there is sensitivity to hot foods, or if there is liver congestion.

Chaparral

A North American Indian herb, this desert plant is one of our greatest and strongest herbal purifiers. The rains in the desert release the fragrance of this plant and the air carries its healing aroma and energy. It is good to use Chaparral during purification programs, and whenever there is arthritis or cancer. It accomplishes a deep level of purification and provides healing to both the urinary system and the lower bowel.

However, if this herb is used over a long period of time it will cleanse too drastically and the patient may feel minor distress from an accumulation of mucus in the alimentary tract in the stomach and throat areas. It is best used in strong doses over a short period of time (for example six capsules three times a day for three weeks), and when combined with an ecological nutrient mix that will allow complete elimination of toxins. Chaparral baths are an excellent way of absorbing the nutrient of this powerful purifier directly into the body through the skin.

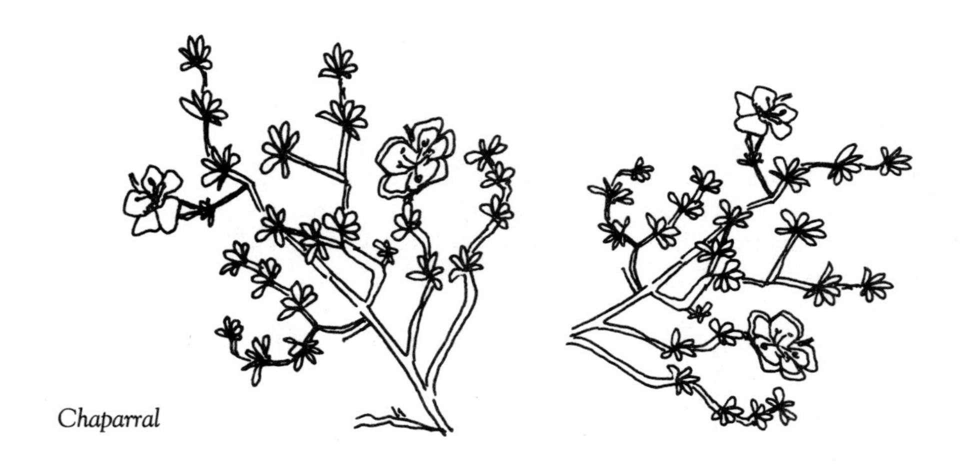

Chaparral

Chickweed

I once had the opportunity to watch the power of Chickweed at work during an acute crisis. Two days after I had seen a new patient who suffered from severe eczema, I received a telephone call early in the morning. She was hysterical from the pain of itching and heat, crying that when she had these crises before she had to be hospitalized, but she did not want to go to the hospital again. I said "Come right over and we'll see what we can do."

By the time she arrived, I had a Chickweed bath waiting and this sobbing, burning, itching woman, quickly climbed into it. Within seconds the heat and the painful itch were relieved. She soaked for a couple of hours and I sent her away with a large bag of Chickweed. For the next few days she either soaked in a Chickweed bath or was wrapped in cloths soaked in Chickweed infusion. To complement the treatment, she fasted on alkaline juices and herbs. She never had a repeat of this terrible crisis. Over the next few months the condition was cleared by systemic purification and rejuvenation. She eventually changed her stressful job at a mental hospital and created a more relaxed way of life to attain complete healing by eliminating the causes.

Use Chickweed internally and externally to relieve itching and help eliminate the acids which cause burning and itching.

Chronic Purifier Formula

This formula provides a deep level of blood, tissue and lymph purification in chronic disease, dyscrasia, syphilis and cancer. Use after the eliminative channels are activated and working efficiently.

Mimosa Gum (2), Echinacea root (3), Blue Flag (3), Comfrey root and Irish Moss

Circulation Cerebral Formula

This formula provides an alternative to the Circulation Systemic formula so that long–term treatment of circulatory disorders do not have to rely on continued use of one formula. Concentrating more on relieving cerebral insufficiency, this formula restores adequate blood flow to the brain areas, relieving tiredness, poor memory, senility and negative mental states.

It is important that it be combined with herbal formulae to discharge morbid accumulations or obstructions in other body areas, organs and systems and to strengthen and support lymph, heart, kidney and liver functions. Every part of the body relies on every other part. When one part of the body is not performing adequately, all the other parts have to adjust and compensate, often to their detriment.

Because poor circulation also affects body temperature and causes the inadequate nourishment of various organs and tissues, it is essential that the circulation be restored if the individual is to regain normal health.

St. John's Wort, Bayberry, Gingko, Prickly Ash, Cayenne and Sage

Circulation Systemic

The herbs that make up this formula increase the range and power of circulation, especially to deficient areas of the body, the extremities and the capillary circulation. This equalization of the circulation restores normal blood pressure, whether high or low. It is especially important to use this formula to carry herbs to deficient areas if the force of circulation is weak or sluggish. Herbal nutrients travel through the blood and the lymph fluids, so it is essential that all areas of the body receive adequate and regular supplies of blood.

Bayberry, Cayenne, Ginger root, Golden Seal root and Hawthorn berries

Colitis Formula

This formula, together with the Bowel Rejuvenator or Bowel Vitalizer, Nerve and Adrenal formulae, works to unravel the complicated causes of this illness. Counseling is also important along with Bach flower remedies to facilitate changes in mental and emotional attitudes and to ensure that the eliminative channels are all working efficiently.

Barberry, Golden Seal root, White Oak bark, Myrrh (0. 25), Slippery Elm and Aniseed

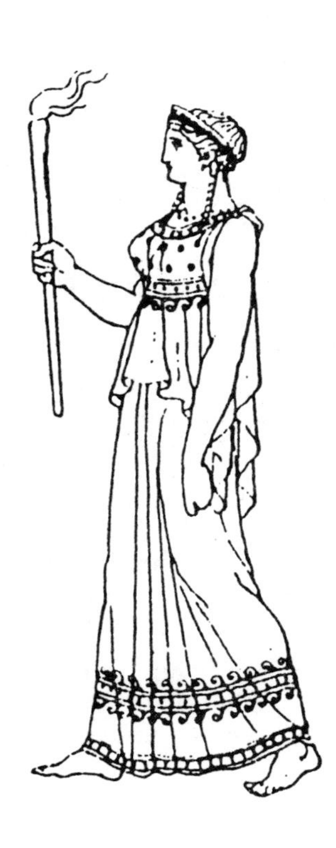

Colds and Flu Formula

This formula, together with the Antibiotics Naturally formula, Mustard baths and sweats relieve uncomfortable symptoms, cleanse the system and ensure a quick healing response without the suppression of toxins caused by the use of medical drugs. Supporting the body's acute responses to eliminate accumulated toxins, these herbal aids and associated acute treatments speed recovery and leave the patient stronger and fitter without laying the ground for the development of chronic disease. Hot Ginger, Yarrow or Ephaedra teas are highly recommended for colds or flu. Use the Sore Throat Syrup described in the Antibiotics Naturally formula section.

Drink Elder flowers and Peppermint tea constantly, day and night. Support the elimination with enemas, Mustard baths and steam under quilts to increase perspiration. Use herbal poultices whenever there are lung, throat or glandular complications.

Elder flowers and Peppermint

Ear Formula

The combination of the antiseptic qualities of Garlic oil together with the ability of Mullein oil to disperse congested lymph glands around the ear, provides an all–around ear treatment which relieves pain, swelling and infection and also improves hearing quality.

Instructions: drop 4 to 6 drops of each oil into the ear every night and morning for six days. Plug the ear with damp cotton batten. Syringe with equal parts of apple cider vinegar and water on the seventh day – about 10 ml. of each. Repeat this seven–day cycle until the condition is relieved. Support with internal herbal treatment for the immune system and also relieve the cause of the infection in the digestive, circulation and lymphatic systems.

Mullein and Garlic oils

Echinacea

This lymphatic herb has a strong and specific power to stimulate lymphatic leukocyte activity. Therefore, its powers for clearing up infection, pus and foul discharges can be used internally and externally wherever tissue decay threatens, or healing repair is slow. It can be added to poultices wherever there is infection. Combine with herbal formulae to activate the eliminative channels and strengthen constitutional weakness. It is important to stop the intake of food, clean the bowels with enemas and drink large quantities of herbal purifying teas whenever there are infections.

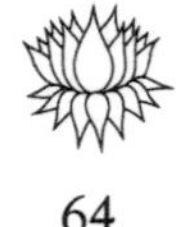

Enema Formula

This formula evolved out of discussions with Margaret Strauss, granddaughter of Dr. Max Gerson, founder of the Gerson Therapy program for cancer and other severe chronic diseases. When I told her about the problems related to adapting their program for strict vegetarian patients, we discussed possible solutions. She clearly felt that if her grandfather had lived longer he would have found vegetarian, herbal substitutions for the coffee enema and the liver and thyroid extracts. She supported the use of my herbal enema formula as an excellent substitute for the coffee enemas.

The added advantage of the herbal enema formula is that superior nutrition is readily available for the direct healing of the walls of the colon, as well as for absorption into the blood and the lymph to be transported throughout the body. After taking this enema one is truly aware of strength and nourishment. The liver is stimulated to dump bile and relieve the system. It also decreases the pain and discomfort of any healing crises.

Instructions: Make a strong decoction by simmering gently one tablespoon Burdock and one tablespoon Yellow Dock root. Turn off the heat. Add one tablespoon Red Clover blossoms and one tablespoon Red Raspberry leaves. Infuse for at least one half hour as it cools. Dilute with distilled water. Inject one quart of the herb mix after the bowel has been cleansed and emptied at least twice with a water enema. Retain five to ten minutes, then expel.

Red Clover blossoms, Red Raspberry leaves, Burdock root and Yellow dock root

Exhaustion Formula

Although exhaustion has many possible causes – mental, emotional and physical – the treatment of this condition usually requires high levels of minerals and vitamins, together with herbs to aid the digestion and assimilation of nutrients and to strengthen and rebuild the adrenal glands and nervous system.

This formula produces excellent recuperative energy to bring clients back to their normal healthy energy level. The Bach flower remedies, *Olive* and *Hornbeam*, and other flower essences are also a great help. Try a Lobelia bath for deep relaxation. Take herbal sedatives such as Lady Slipper and Valerian. Sleep and rest. Take Chamomile aromatherapy baths and polarity therapy, acupuncture, cranial sacral, shiatsu and reflexology to release stress and tension.

Above all, take a good look at life style. Living in the fast lane and creating burn–out and stress is asking for trouble. Exhaustion is the body calling out for help and change. Its time to break old patterns. Take a vacation, or stay home and sleep all weekend.

You may feel your exhaustion more when you begin taking the herbal nutrients because your true level of energy is revealed. You can no longer push beyond your limits or ignore your body. During the healing period it is essential to take extra time to rest and sleep, and to curtail all non–essential activities. Discontinue taking any stimulants or caffeine.

Gentian root (2), Gotu Kola (2), Chondrus Crispus, Cetraria, Alfalfa and Calumba root

Eye Wash Formula

This eye wash has been successfully used by herbalists for many years for the treatment of cataract, glaucoma, eye weakness and infection. The herbs stimulate circulation to the eyes, relieve congestion, nourish the eyes and cure infection. Although there is sometimes mild stinging when first using the eye wash, this soon passes and the eyes feel bright, refreshed and strengthened. Use one eighth teaspoon of the herb to one half cup water.

Pour boiling water over the herbal powder, steep until it cools, and then strain well through a fine cloth or coffee filter. Using an eye cup, open and close each eye under the infusion for at least one minute. Do this once, twice or three times a day as needed, and continue until the condition is improved. If the eyes are particularly sensitive, dilute the strained infusion further.

Eyebright and Golden Seal root

Female Reproductive Formula

This herbal combination strengthens, tones, regulates and heals the reproductive organs. Whatever the problem or symptoms, this formula provides the nutrients to support regeneration. It is essential that the eliminative channels be fully cleansed and activated, and that systemic weaknesses are supported if long–term healing is to be achieved. This formula works deeply, relieving cramps, menstrual flooding and pain, and prepares the female reproductive system for healthy childbearing. Combine this formula with the Women's Period Pain formula when cramps and lower backache accompany monthly periods. Combine it with the Menopause or Hormone formulae during the change of life.

Blue Cohosh, Licorice root, Motherwort, Parsley root, Red Raspberry leaves, Squaw Vine and True Unicorn root

Fenugreek

The highest vegetable source of vitamin D, Fenugreek supports skin rejuvenation programs. Whenever the skin is not eliminating properly, perspiration is insufficient, or the skin is dry and scaly, take six to eight cups of Fenugreek tea a day, one level teaspoon of powder per cup, or simmer the seeds very gently for fifteen minutes and drink throughout the day. The Fenugreek can also be taken in powder or tincture form. This stimulates perspiration and increases gentle elimination. Shower and bathe more often during this treatment, as the skin will eliminates acids and toxins. Take an Epsom salts and cider vinegar bath every other day. After bathing rub the skin with a mixture of almond and wheat germ oil, and scrub the skin twice daily with a natural bristle brush.

Fungus/Candida Formula

Although most cases clear during constitutional, eliminative and systemic treatments, when combined with the vaginal ovule and douche, this formula is useful when fungal infections on fingers, feet or elsewhere prove resistant. This formula augments any total approach to clearing the system while helping to relieve irritating symptoms. Use internally and externally as a poultice, bath or douche.

For best results, do not mix herbs or formulae containing seaweeds with this formula as iodine neutralizes the action.

Thyme, Poke root, Myrrh, Cleavers, Cayenne and Meadowsweet

Gall Bladder Formula

This formula completes the gall bladder cleanse as outlined in the Herbal and Naturopathy Treatments chapter. It should be taken for at least six weeks after the cleanse to reduce inflammation and strengthen and heal the gall bladder.

Black root, Euonymous, Kava Kava and Marshmallow root (2)

Gentian

This root is added to eliminative and systemic treatment whenever the absorption of nutrient, digestive weakness or exhaustion are major problems. A strengthening and revitalizing herb, Gentian tones the liver and makes an effective digestive tonic.

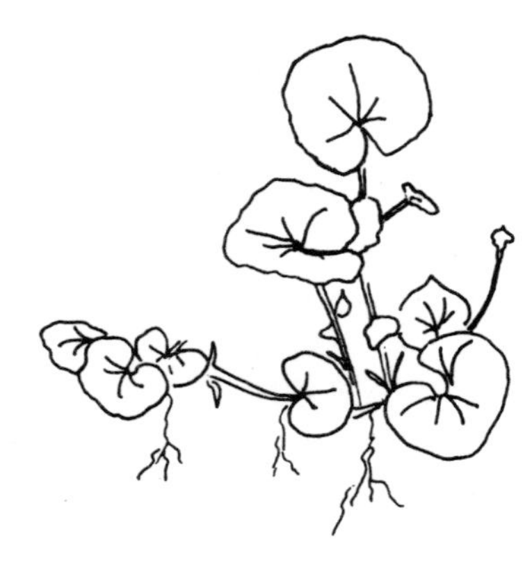

Gotu Kola

Gotu Kola

An effective nerve restorative and mental soother, this herb is mixed in equal parts with Calamus when the digestive and nervous systems require combined treatment.

Hair Strengthening Formula

When hair is weak, brittle or falling out, use this formula to complement systemic treatment. It is essential that the Circulation formula together with purifying herbs also be used to improve the absorption and assimilation of nutrients and their circulation to the head.

Make an herbal tea of Sage, Yarrow and Yellow Dock, using one tablespoon of each herbal powder to one cup of water. Wash the hair while the tea is steeping and then massage it into the hair and scalp. Do not rinse out. Leave it on all day.

In the evening make a mixture of equal parts of Castor oil, wheat germ oil and olive oil, and massage into the head and hair. Steam with hot towels, wrap in a dry towel and leave on all night. Wash the hair well in the morning and then massage in the herb tea again. Leave it on all day. During the day practice inversion postures or slant board exercises. Drink Sage tea, take one or both of the Circulation formulae, and take high doses of vitamin E. Continue this treatment for a full seven week cycle and repeat at regular intervals for best results.

Sage, Yarrow and Yellow Dock root

Heart Tonic Formula

This normalizing heart formula improves blood pressure, eliminates water retention, strengthens the heart rate, clears arterial deposits, equalizes the force of heart contractions, increases peripheral circulation and beneficially influences the nervous system, providing a wide range of nutrients to balance, strengthen and nourish this hardworking organ. Combine with either or both of the Circulation formulae for best results.

Hawthorn berries (6), Motherwort (3), Ginseng root (3), Ginger root (2), Comfrey root (2), Lily of the Valley (3), Broom (2), Dandelion leaves(2), Scullcap (2), Lime blossoms (2) and Bugleweed (2)

Heavy Metal Purifier Formula

After a certain level of eliminative function and systemic balance has been achieved on a six to eight week purification and rejuvenation program, this formula can be given to release a deeper level of cleansing. However, it is essential that all the eliminative channels are working well or the patient will experience headaches, nausea and weakness.

It is important that this formula be combined with the Kidney/Bladder formula, taken on its own between meals with a glass of water or herb tea. Daily Epsom salt baths will increase elimination from the skin. The Heavy Metal formula stimulates the release of toxins which need to be eliminated from the bowels, kidneys, skin, lymph and lungs.

This formula will slowly reduce the shape and size of iris pigmentation markings. Take it over a three week period, rest three weeks, then repeat. The Heavy Metal formula reaches deeply into the tissues to release toxins which have collected in weak areas. If the treatment is guided properly there should be neither discomfort nor weakness as purification progresses.

Yellow Dock root, Bugleweed, Lobelia, Chaparral and Uva Ursi

HORMONE BALANCE FORMULA

The herbs in this formula contain natural hormones offered within complex plant chemistry so that the patients, whether male or female, will be provided with both estrogen and progesterone. The individual body will select what is needed for balance. Use confidently during pregnancy, puberty or menopause, or whenever endocrine functions need tuning.

Black Cohosh root, Sarsaparilla, Ginseng root, Holy Thistle, Licorice root, False Unicorn root, Squaw Vine and Chasteberry

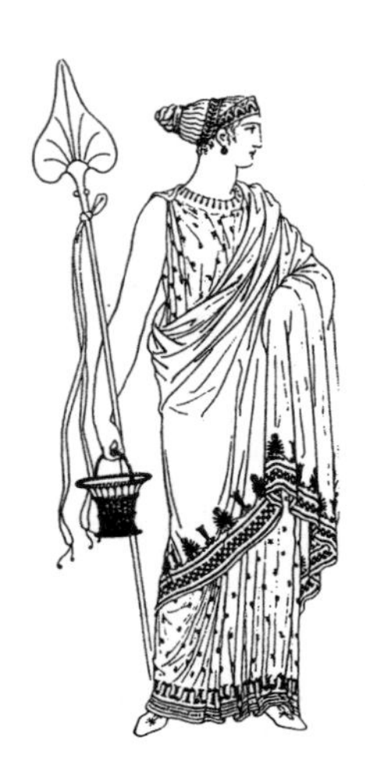

HYDRANGEA

Once one of our British School of iridology graduates was hospitalized with severe kidney pains. After undergoing several days of tests and treatments without improvement and considerable pain, he discharged himself and applied the Hydrangea root treatment. After passing a kidney stone with relative ease, he was cleared of all pain with no recurrence. However, his other eliminative systems were functioning well due to his natural life style. Preparation of the eliminative channels, body organs and systems to a level of active function increases the effectiveness of this treatment. I also advise using the Castor oil pack over the abdomen and the Ginger poultice over the kidneys for at least three days before attempting this treatment. Full instructions are given in the Kidney and Gall Stone Cleanse in the Herbal and Naturopathiy Treatments chapter. Use a strong decoction of Hydrangea root to dissolve calcareous kidney stones. Take at least four to six cups daily for seven weeks while following a purification diet and systemic internal herbal treatment guided by an Iridologist.

Individuals have varying tolerances for Hydrangea root, or any specific herb taken in high doses over a length of time. If there are any minor aggravations or signs of toxicity building up, use kineseology or radionics to determine the maximum dose and the length of time to take the Hydrangea root to dissolve the stones. Monitor the dose by being sensitive to body changes and reducing the dose as required. Our program of balanced treatment minimizes such aggravations, but it is always wise to be sensitive, as each person is so individual.

Ileocaecal Valve Formula

This formula regulates over–functioning or under–functioning ileocaecal imbalances. Chiropractors, osteopaths, polarity therapists or applied kineseology practitioners can help to release and adjust this valve. They are also educated about its influence on the digestive system, and the mental and emotional stresses and tensions which aggravate ileocaecal problems. It is essential to treat the nervous system and the adrenals, and take either of the Bowel formulae. Abdominal Castor oil packs will also help to relieve symptoms. Lie on the back with the knees up and massage the psoas muscle on either side of the abdomen to release tension.

Ginger root(0.5), Quassia, Bistort, Bayberry and Angelica root

Infection Formula

Acute infections require high doses of herbs to stimulate the lymphatic system to deal with the invasion. Keep this formula on hand in your first aid kit. For acute infections administer four to six capsules every half hour. Reduce to two capsules for children under twelve years, one capsule for children under seven, and one half capsule for children under two years of age.

This formula is useful for the treatment of colds, flu, fever, abscesses, infected wounds, bronchitis and burns. It is best to have the guidance of a doctor in any serious condition, and certainly if natural medicines are to be used, it is essential that the bowels and stomach are clean and clear. Fast on juices and drink copious amounts of herbal teas.

Whenever there are fevers, clear the bowels with Catnip enemas, soak in a very hot Mustard bath as long as possible, and follow by resting under several blankets in a bed packed with hot water bottles. This encourages a free flow of perspiration, which relieves the system. It is important to stay under the quilts until the body has returned to normal temperature. Drink Yarrow tea during the bath to increase perspiration, and follow with copious amounts of Red Raspberry, Catnip and Peppermint tea during and after perspiring under the quilts. After the body has cooled, sponge with equal parts of apple cider vinegar and water, and dress in warm cotton clothes. It is beneficial to exercise gently indoors or outdoors, but if there is weakness or sensitivity, return to bed. Clients report that symptoms clear, the fever is reduced quickly and they feel quite well on recovery, without lingering weakness.

Echinacea root (2), Garlic, Golden Seal root, Lobelia, Mullein and Plantain

Intestinal Infection Formula

This formula can be used with bowel cleansing, or to clear intestinal infections from tropical climates. It helps to eliminate harmful microbial parasites and infections in bowel pockets and diverticuli. Although its influence is strong, it is important to have medical tests and consult a doctor or practitioner. Eat large amounts of pumpkin seeds daily (whole or freshly powdered in a coffee grinder) until the condition is cleared. Herbal enemas are also effective.

Gentian root, Burdock root, Wormwood(2), Sage, Fennel, Mullein, Myrrh, Thyme (2) and Quassia

Kidney/Bladder Formula

This formula cleanses, heals and balances urine flow, dissolves sediment, tones, and strengthens the function of the entire urinary tract. Kidney problems are not always directly due to kidney weakness. The kidneys also suffer because of the lack of support from other eliminative channels, or because of improper drinking habits. Within the framework of systemic and eliminative treatment, this formula brings the function of the urinary tract to a healthy balanced level.

Buchu, Clivers, Gravel root, Juniper berries, Marshmallow root, Parsley root and Uva Ursi

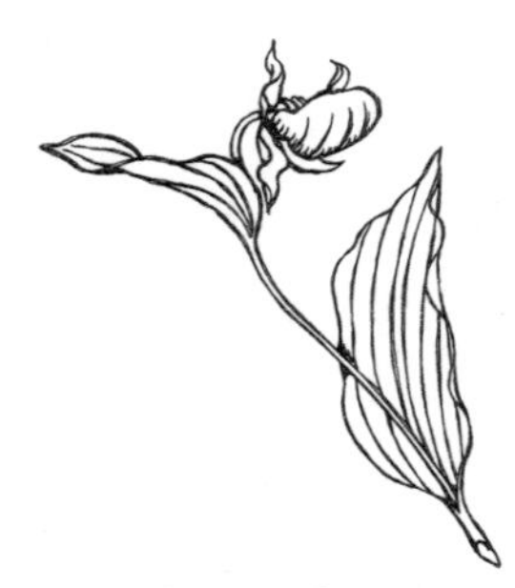

Lady Slipper

One of my favorite herbs, Lady Slipper root is a cerebral sedative that breaks the pattern of stress and strain, gives excellent sleep and relieves emotional sensitivity. It provides a fresh start in the morning, producing a relaxed state which is a relief to any nervous system wound up by work, family or personal crises. It is an excellent aid for jet travel, allowing total relaxation and releasing anxious tensions during the flight, so that travellers arrive fresh and rested. This is a prime remedy for individuals whose illnesses stem from the nervous system. When balance is restored by a complete rest and good sleep, the system does not suffer a breakdown of health.

Lady Slipper, now an endangered alpine orchid, is no longer readily available for use individually or in formulae. Valerian is the next best alternative, but for those who can propagate their own supplies of Lady Slipper, their efforts will prove worthwhile.

Dosage: from three to twelve capsules, before sleep or while travelling, depending on the person's age, size, condition and circumstances.

LADY SLIPPER/VALERIAN

This combination reduces the expense of using pure Lady Slipper and it is also more suitable for those who run on their nerves during the day and are restless and unable to sit down or stop doing things. Divide into three daily doses of two to four capsules per dose. This formula prepares the body to withdraw from tranquilizers or relaxants, and it can also be used before sleep to ensure a good night's rest.

Lady's Slipper root and Valerian root

LIVER/GALL BLADDER FORMULA

The digestive chemical factory needs the full support of liver and gall bladder functions to secrete the alkaline fluids into the duodenum that balance the acid secretions from the pancreas. Together they act on the food that comes from the stomach. This formula begins its work in the stomach and proceeds to influence the digestive process of the liver because it deals with the metabolism of carbohydrates, proteins, fats and the storage and metabolism of vitamins. A healthy liver means clean blood and a good digestion, essential aspects of optimum body function.

The liver also has a strong emotional association with passionate anger, aggression, jealousy and power struggles. It is wise to explore these aggravations and include Bach flower remedies and counseling in holistic treatment.

Barberry bark (3), Wild Yam root, Cramp bark, Fennel, Catnip, Peppermint, Dandelion root(2), Meadowsweet (2), Wahoo and Black root

LYMPHATIC FORMULA

Whenever the lymph system is constitutionally deficient (indicated by a lymphatic rosary in the iris), it is unable to deal with further levels of catarrh created by incorrect diet, high levels of toxins, or invasion by viruses or germs. This formula strengthens and activates the leukocytes, supports the lymph glands, and stimulates balanced elimination. It is important to first consider the level of toxins and the functioning of the other eliminative channels and blood purifying organs, such as the liver and the kidneys, and add appropriate additional formulae as required. Alternate with the Chronic Purifier formula for best results.

Echinacea root, Lobelia, Mullein, Poke root, Burdock root, Cayenne and Chaparral

Menopause Formula

Although every woman and her experience of menopause is unique, this formula offers a background of nourishment, and support for more specific treatment. As well as balancing hormones this formula offers superior nourishment, including natural calcium to help avoid bone loss. It strengthens the kidneys and adrenals, supports the liver and digestive system, relieves hot flashes, eases sore joints and increases energy.

Alfalfa, Chickweed, Dandelion root, Dong Quai, Fenugreek, Horsetail, Motherwort, Nettles, Red Clover blossoms, Red Raspberry leaves, Violet leaves and Wild Yam root

Milk Thistle

The seeds of this herb can be used to great advantage whenever there is poisoning, chronic skin disease and liver disorders. Add this herb to any program for psoriasis, eczema or liver regeneration. It can also be made into juice from fresh seeds or into powder from dried seeds.

Mucus Congestion Formula

This natural antihistamine relieves irritating sinus and nasal problems associated with colds, flu and hay fever and reduces uncomfortable mucus elimination. Use in combination with the Antibiotics Naturally or the Infection formulae.

Black Pepper, Aniseed and Ginger root

Mullein

Diarrhea can be a severe problem during bowel illness and bowel rejuvenation programs. It is essential to use a combination of treatments to reduce the diarrhea as quickly as possible because it is so uncomfortable and debilitating. Mullein tea mixed with hot water or soy milk reduces diarrhea. In stubborn cases also eat a diet of stewed apples with high amounts of cinnamon, baked potatoes and Slippery Elm tea. Astringent enemas or rectal injections of Red Raspberry, Witch Hazel or Bayberry infusions are also useful.

Multi–Minerals/Vitamins Naturally Formula

This is a superior balanced herbal alternative to mineral and vitamin supplements! Although our fresh, potent, unprocessed herbal nutrients are richly endowed with vitamins and minerals, this formula contains the full range – a great saving when prices are compared with processed vitamin/mineral supplements. It also contains easily assimilable vegetarian alkaline protein and amino acids. Adjust dose according to need. Two teaspoons provide the equivalent nutrients of a meal and help to take away hunger pangs during healing diets or cleansing fasts.

Alfalfa, Alkaline formula(4), Anemia formula, Calcium formula(2), Spirulina and Rose hips

Nerve Rejuvenator Formula

This formula restores the nervous system and encourages deep rejuvenating sleep. Take regularly throughout the day as well as six to eight capsules when needed before sleep. It helps rebuild the nervous system after mental or emotional nervous breakdowns.

Gotu Kola (4), Valerian root (2), Kava Kava, Irish Moss and Lady Slipper root

Nerve Tonic Formula

Rebuilding the nervous system requires regular intake of nervine herbs, which provide the nutrient for central, autonomic and peripheral nervous systems. Combine this formula with the Calcium, Sweet Sleep or Thyroid formulae if there are problems with hyperactivity or insomnia.

Catnip, Gotu Kola (2), Lady's Slipper root, Lobelia, Scullcap and Valerian root

Nerve Vitalizer Formula

This formula strengthens the nervous system during and after trauma, shock, extreme stress, fatigue and accidents.

Prickly Ash bark (4), Irish Moss and Bayberry bark

Pain Relief Formula

Whether pain is from acute injuries, headaches, burns, or from chronic diseases like arthritis and rheumatism, this formula will soothe, diminish the discomfort, and encourage sleep. The dose can be adjusted from three times a day with meals to every fifteen minutes, one–half hour, or every hour as needed. It works best in combination with professionally guided treatment to relieve the cause of the pain. Dosage: one to four capsules as needed.

White Willow bark, Jamaican Dogwood, Valerian root and Cramp bark

Pancreas Formula

The herbs in this formula offer natural insulin that helps to lower blood sugar levels and strengthen and feed this gland. Use this formula as part of a holistic systemic program. Hypoglycemia will also be relieved by this formula, especially if several cups of Licorice tea are drunk throughout the day. Eat vegetarian, alkaline, fresh organic food and fresh juices.

Elecampagne (2), Golden Seal root, Uva Ursi, Wahoo (2), Licorice root, Mullein, Nettles, Allspice and Juniper berries

Pre–Natal Formula

The expectant mother should drink several cups of this tea during the last six weeks of pregnancy to aid the elasticity of the birth canal and strengthen the reproductive organs for easier delivery. It is also good to take regular doses of the Calcium and Anemia formulae throughout the entire pregnancy and while nursing. These are purely nutritive herbs which should not upset the mother or the baby. Blue Cohosh root decoction or tincture may be taken from the early stages of labor to the birth to ease and relax the birth canal and to minimize pain.

Holy Thistle, Red Raspberry, Squaw Vine and True Unicorn

Prolapse Formula

There are many factors which contribute to a prolapsed colon condition. The case history and iridology reading will help to determine whether it is related to weak connective tissue, pressure from other organs, bowel toxins or nutritional deficiency. Internal herbal treatment can be supported by specific feeding of the pelvic area by the use of ovules and douches. Refer to the Herbal and Naturopathy Treatments chapter.

Black Cohosh, Witch Hazel, White Oak bark (2), Lobelia, Yellow Dock and Marshmallow root

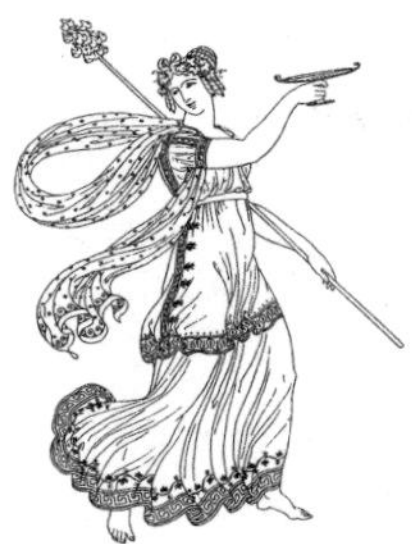

Prostate Formula

Combine this formula with the Bowel Rejuvenator and Lymphatic formulae. Take over a period of eight weeks to strengthen this gland. Use the rectal ovule as well. Refer to the Vagina/Prostrate ovule treatment in the Herbal and Naturopathy Treatments chapter.

Echinacea root, Saw Palmetto berries, Gravel root, Parsley root, Golden Seal root(2), Marshmallow root and Cayenne

Psyllium

Soak one teaspoon of Psyllium seeds in one–half cup of warm water. Add juice to improve the taste if you wish. This mucilaginous mixture sweeps the bowel walls clean and provides bulk to ease constipation. Take concurrently with either of the Bowel formulae, during a bowel cleanse treatment, but do not use on a regular long–term basis.

Respiratory Formula

This formula supports the respiratory system when it is actively eliminating, infected or chronically weak from conditions like asthma and bronchitis. It works best when it is combined with the Asthma formula, as well as systemic treatment for activating and cleansing the eliminative channels and purifying and regenerating the body systems and organs.

Comfrey root, Elecampagne, Elder flowers, Mullein (2), Licorice root and Lobelia

Skin Problems Formula

Chronic skin problems are deep–seated and involve all the blood purifying organs, the eliminative channels and the defense systems of the skin itself. This deeply purifying formula works well in combination with systemic treatment to eliminate morbid conditions from the blood that cause the skin to suffer the consequences. It is also essential to improve the diet. Add the following to the program: the Bowel Rejuvenator, Liver/Gall Bladder, and Kidney/Bladder formulae, and Milk Thistle seeds.

Blue Flag, Burdock root, Burdock seeds, Cayenne, Echinacea root, Poke root and Red Clover blossoms

Slippery Elm

Whenever a sensitive digestive system reacts against food or herbs, Slippery Elm forms the perfect carrier to reduce discomfort. Make a warm drink of one teaspoon Slippery Elm powder with one cup of warm soy milk or water, and add honey, maple syrup, Carob or Cinnamon as desired to improve the taste. Mix and drink immediately, before it becomes too thick. As well as soothing and protecting the intestinal wall and easing digestion, this herbal nutrient is a highly nutritious food which contains abundant calcium.

This mucilaginous herb is also used with poultices and the vaginal ovule because it helps to hold the herbal powders together.

Smoking Formula

This formula reduces the need for nicotine, alters taste cravings so that the desire for smoking is reduced and relieves pain in the respiratory system. I have known many patients who have completely stopped smoking after using this mix. Roll into a handmade herbal 'cigarette' and smoke!

The smoking mix is also excellent for relieving respiratory pain in chronic lung diseases. The Lobelia relaxes the chest and disperses congestion, while the Mullein soothes, heals and comforts. Lobelia poultices are an excellent complement to this treatment.

Coltsfoot, Mullein, Yerba Santa and Lobelia

Spirulina

This nutritious algae contains almost every mineral and vitamin required in our diet, including a high amount of B vitamins and assimilable alkaline protein. Whenever there is weakness, exhaustion, strong cravings or hunger, this food helps to balance digestion. It is an excellent supplement to use during fasts, juice cleanses and purifying diets.

Stomach Acid/Alkaline Balancing Formula

Imbalances of body chemistry often begin in the stomach. Whether the stomach is too acid or too alkaline this formula will provide the wide range of nutrients necessary to normalize the stomach environment. It is also useful to add this formula wherever the digestion is sensitive because it helps soothe and heal the stomach and ease other herbs into the system.

Dandelion root, Slippery Elm, Calamus, Meadowsweet, Irish Moss and Iceland Moss

Sweet Sleep Formula

Restful sleep depends to a large extent on the ability of our parasympathetic nervous system to relax and release us from the stress and strain of daily activities. These herbs mildly sedate the nervous system and encourage a sweet restful sleep that leaves one rested, yet alert in the morning. During times of stress or intense activity, this formula can also be taken with food at regular intervals during the day.

Passion flowers, Lady Slipper root, Valerian root, Scullcap, Hops, Broom and Lime tree flowers

Swollen Glands Formula

Use this formula internally, and as a fomentation to relieve congestion and reduce swelling and discomfort. Use with the Lymphatic and Antibiotics Naturally formulae for best results. Leave the fomentation on all night and day if necessary, six days a week.

Lobelia, Mullein (2), Parsley root or leaves and Plantain

Tableting Formula

Use with tableting rollers and cutters, or for hand–rolled tablets. This formula will reduce sticking and finish the tablets with a tasty nutritive powder. Sprinkle carob on the tablets to further improve the taste.

Alkaline formula (2), Slippery Elm and Cinnamon or Carob

Thyroid Balancing Formula

Whether the thyroid is underactive or overactive, the body, mind and emotions become disturbed if this master gland does not receive the nutrients required for balanced activity. Use this formula together with the Adrenal, Sweet Sleep, or Nerve formulae for an overactive thyroid, or with the Exhaustion and Multi–Mineral formulae if the thyroid is underactive.

Parsley leaves, Kelp (2), Irish Moss, Iceland Moss, Nettles, Bladderwrack and Bugleweed

VAGINAL/PROSTATE OVULE FORMULA

The vaginal ovule is an internal poultice which is used to transform the environment of the vagina, to offer superior healing nutrition and to draw out toxic poisons from the tissues, blood and lymph. Although the deeper cause may be inherited, or the result of mental, emotional and living influences combined with systemic toxicity, much can be gained by using the ovule locally to relieve chronic reproductive conditions, discharges, irritation, itching and sores. The ovule also positively influences deeper conditions such as cysts, tumors, inflammation, sores and cervical dysplasia, providing nutrients for healing exactly where they are needed.

The herbs are absorbed into the mucus membranes and spread via the capillary circulation and lymph into the pelvis. When the ovule is supported with herbal nutrients taken internally, the influences meet, contributing to total healing. Visualize the pelvis as an environment where everything touches everything else, where either toxins or healing can spread out from the bowels through the circulation of lymph and blood. Emotional and muscular tensions in the solar plexus also inhibit peristalsis. If healing is to take place the pelvis must be cleansed and restored to harmonious function within the total ecology of the whole person. Please refer to the Herbal and Naturopathy Treatments chapter for specific instructions.

Squaw Vine, Echinacea root, Comfrey root, Marshmallow root, Chickweed and Golden Seal root

WILD YAM

Whenever flatulence, gas, wind, spasms, colic or stomach discomfort contribute strong symptoms, this root is added to the herbal nutrient mix. It is also excellent for uterine cramps. It can be taken together with the Women's Period Pain formula throughout pregnancy both as a tonic and to prevent miscarriage. This herb is also a natural source of progesterone precursors and has applications for women's reproductive and hormonal conditions and menopause.

WOMEN'S PERIOD PAIN FORMULA

If cramps and pain disturb your menstrual cycle, use this formula just before your period is due and during any discomfort. Because the effect is accumulative, the need for it should lessen from month to month, especially if the causes are being relieved by systemic purification and rejuvenation. Chamomile tea will also help relieve cramps when it is taken immediately.

Blue Cohosh, Cramp bark (2), Lemon Balm, Ginger root, Turmeric and Valerian root

YELLOW DOCK

Yellow Dock root is used for the douche which supports the Vaginal ovule treatment. Its high iron content attracts oxygen, increases cellular metabolism and restores health to the mucus membrane. It is also part of the Anemia formula which is taken throughout pregnancy. An herbal decoction made from the root or tea made from powdered root are excellent ways to take iron in an easily assimilable form. A valuable blood–purifying herb and a lymphatic stimulant, Yellow Dock contributes a positive influence whenever it is used.

5

Nourishment

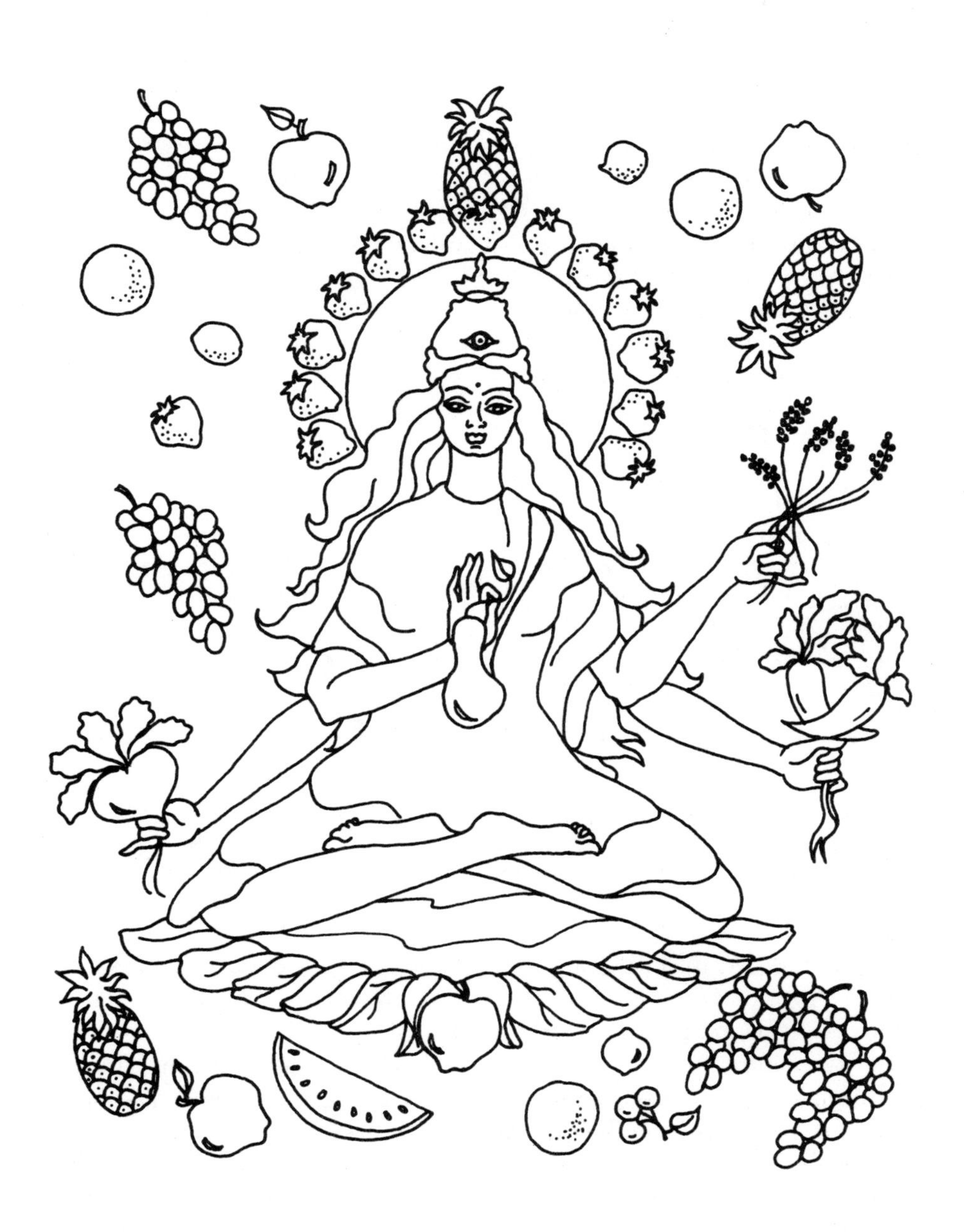

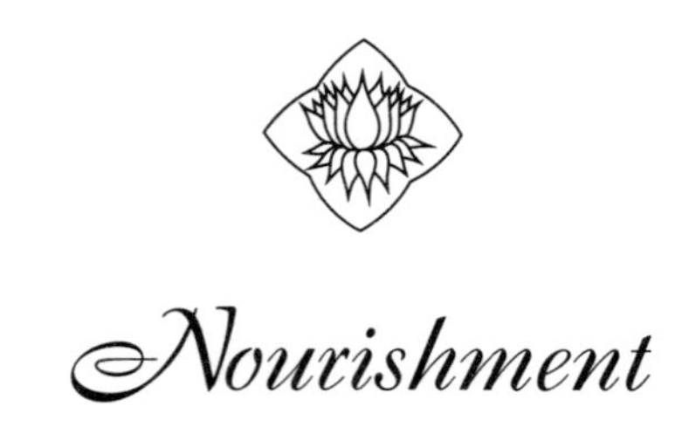

Nourishment

This chapter explores the meaning of nourishment and includes diets which complement the herbal nutrients and home treatments. It presents the information needed to maintain health on a daily basis and to clear any acute problems that may arise. There is much we can do to prevent illness and achieve healing.

Although ideal diets are described here, humans are not ideal. We make efforts, gradually adjust, and strive to improve our living habits. It is important to approach purification as a transition, slowly and comfortably. Read. Think. Experiment. Experience foods and drinks that are good for us. We need to retrain ourselves to enjoy what is wholesome, natural, nutritious and healthy. We must make a place for delight and pleasure in practical and pleasant ways. We can create attractive meals with fresh, organic foods and use the senses to appreciate the beauty of food that is alive and vibrant.

Dietary changes are supported by herbal nutrients that create a foundation of strength and energy. Within this framework of support, dietary changes and improvements are naturally eased into daily life. After the herbal treatment is completed the improved diet will keep positive changes moving ahead.

Strictness, denial and rigidity about new dietary habits will create negative digestion just as much as unhappiness, anger, stress and worry. Don't think about what is being given up. Think of what is being received. As the body adjusts, tastes and cravings diminish. If we really want to eat something, let's enjoy it, and then watch and see how it agrees with us. Indulgence can also teach us lessons. Treats are an important part of life, but we should not eat treats at every meal. If we persevere with good living habits, the day will come when we will want the foods that are good for us. That is health.

Nourishment is the essence of life. Our relationship with the divine, our parents, family, society and this world is all based on receiving, or not receiving, the nourishment we need in every realm of being. We go through life believing that we choose what nourishes us, what makes us happy, and what we think is good for us. Yet, when we are ill, unbalanced, ignorant, deprived, unconscious or rebellious, we often choose what will poison us, hurt us or set us further off balance. For over twenty years I have observed how clients' diet, drink, living habits and personal relationships were toxic to their body, emotions, mind and life. It is as though their ability to recognize positive nourishment had been lost, so they chose short–term addictions, stimulation and strong tastes even though they knew these foods and drinks were hurting them and aggravating their health problems. Some people do not even realize the connection between their foods and drinks and their health condition.

In a sense, our relationship with nourishment begins even before conception, when our life pattern connects with the life pattern of our parents, and we become part of their positivity and their negativity in this realm of duality. As we are conceived from the energy of our parents and formed within their sexual relationship, their patterns of nourishment are passed on to us. Birth, our reception into the world, touching, talking, feeling and nursing form our primal ground of nourishment, which continues through infancy, childhood, puberty and maturity.

We learn how to ask for what we want, and we either get what we want or we don't. We watch those around us work, suffer, manipulate, steal, lie and seduce what they want out of the world, and we learn what gets results. Our personality forms around our ability to deal with acceptance or refusal. We have dreams, goals and ideas that we believe will give us what we want and nourish us and satisfy us, but most often when we attain them we find we are still hungry. This sense of emptiness, deprivation and starvation is strong even in the wealthiest families. How often do we feel truly nourished in every aspect of our being – content, relaxed and at peace? This spiritually evolved state is rare. Most of us live our lives seeking nourishment and stimulation. Our highs are only temporary. For most of us hunger is our life experience.

Our patterns of food and drink revolve around hunger, desire, emptiness and longing that are actually reflections of spiritual separation and the need for true nourishment. Very few of us eat food as food. We eat and taste to satisfy emotional cravings and we eat too much, too fast. We substitute processed, indulgent, junk or fad foods for nutritive foods. Whether we eat too much or too little, we often eat to show that we are wealthy, in style, elegant, powerful, seductive or creative. We also eat as we close business deals, during interviews, as we work, and during power struggles with family members. We also eat on the run, while driving cars, or watching television or movies and standing up. How many of us eat the right amount of simple foods in a relaxed manner, enjoying good company and laughter?

Time and again clients tell me that when they were young nearly every meal at the family table was a power struggle of argument and upset. Food became associated with stomach cramps, anxiety and fear. Thousands of case histories have revealed the most bizarre eating and drinking habits. As clients describe their daily patterns they begin to get a glimmer of how they are creating their illness. Addictions to soda beverages, burritos, chips and salsa, bread, sugar, alcohol, coffee, tea, salt and chocolate are combined with habits like gulping down food, not chewing, eating fruit with meat, drinking glasses of iced water with meals, overeating, throwing up after eating, or eating nothing but meat or eggs or rice. It is amazing what people do.

It is time to take a good long look at what you do with food and drink. How do you feel when you sit down to a meal? Do you take time to lovingly create a beautiful meal for yourself? Do you feel good after you eat? Are you influenced by others? Do you live on snacks? What tastes are you addicted to? Do you use stimulants? What foods cause reactions? Do you have allergies? When did they start? What was happening in your life when the addictions or allergies started?

Putting food into one end of the gastrointestinal tract is only part of the picture. Difficulties can be experienced at any stage of the journey, and how and what is released from the other end through bowel matter and urine tells the remainder of the story. We must change the journey of our food from the moment our mind thinks of it, to the first response of emotional and taste craving, to how we prepare, eat, digest, assimilate and eliminate. We must change the journey of our food to one of true nourishment. It is important to learn how to make the journey of our nourishment a healthy, happy one.

Food can be food or poison or medicine. This chapter is about food as medicine. Food can bring us back into balance when it is truly nourishment, given to oneself by oneself, consciously from self–love, not as a vehicle for addiction, cravings, or emotional starvation and hunger.

Any evaluation of nourishment patterns creates the opportunity for new positive patterns that will bring health, energy and joy into life. When we realize that every choice we make with regard to food and drink creates not only the physical body but the quality of emotion, the ability of mind to function in different ways, and vibratory resonance with spirituality and with other living beings, it will be easier to participate consciously in every decision we make.

We need to use our personal situations, skills and strengths to help us change our nourishment patterns. If we are in the business world we can use strategies, long–term planning and administrative abilities to achieve our health goals. Housewives can use their freedom, time and skills to focus on health while managing their households. Students can use natural healing to help them achieve higher grades and prepare for their future careers. We must use whatever skills and abilities we possess to include natural preventive living and medicine into our lives. We must learn to take care of our health as well as our car, home or business. We must not sacrifice our health to attain our goals. We must not spend the first half of our lives creating problems that will ruin the positive possibilities of our elder years and retirement.

We must say yes to what will give us health and positive energy, and say no to what will cause future health problems. We may think we are only paying the cost of an indulgent meal and the accompanying wines, liquors, cigarettes and desserts, but the meal should also include the cost of hospitalization, insurance and loss of work that future health problems will bring into our lives. The quality of our lives is an even greater reason to take positive control over our decisions. Eliminate the old and bring in the new.

The lives we live in our bodies is our experiment with our inner and outer worlds. When our pattern of cause and effect produces disease, it is time to change our experiment and make that pattern conscious. We must create a relationship of true nourishment between our inner being and the world around us. What we choose to eat affects our health, other living creatures and our relationship with our loved ones, family, friends, community, country and world. As we make positive enlightened choices we will clear confusion from our nourishment patterns.

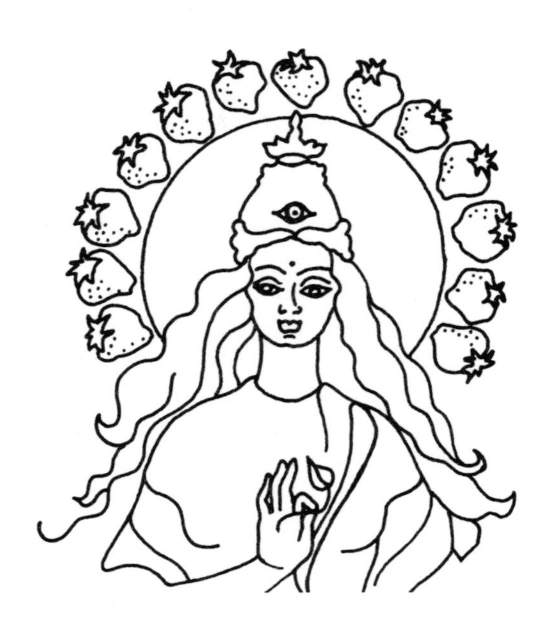

BREAKING ADDICTIONS, CRAVINGS AND NEGATIVE FOOD HABITS

Changing deep patterns of nutritional imbalances requires patience, perseverance, effort and support. Getting fed up and angry at what we have been doing can be a great motivating force. We can use the energy of the digestive fire element for transformation. The support of herbal nutrients combined with dietary changes, home treatments, exercise and flower essences ease the way. As the eliminative systems clear, activate and regenerate, body, emotions, mind and spirit experience relief. Energy begins to move, and positive changes unfold.

Every poison food that is replaced with a medicine food will contribute to healing progress. When tastes for excessive amounts of salt, sugar, spices, coffee and alcohol are discontinued, the taste buds begin to normalize and further relieve addictions and cravings. The desire to binge can be redirected through exercise, counseling, bowel cleansing and body work.

Our greatest creation is our own life. As we grow from the roots of infancy and childhood through the stemming and leafing of puberty and early adulthood to the flowering, fruiting and seeding of maturity and old age, we realize we must not waste this opportunity. Discipline, strength, vision, purpose, perseverance and willingness should decorate our table, refrigerator and kitchen shelves. Our body is a reflection of who we are. The food we eat, and how we eat it, create who we will become.

We are what we eat, and we eat what we are. We must make our food choices conscious, and reach for the highest and the best forms of nourishment, so that we can experience true satisfaction, health, peace and contentment.

For example, if we have been drinking twenty cups of coffee a day and need to stop, the answer is not to say no and suffer, but to approach this problem in a practical and positive way. Excessive cravings reflect imbalances within. The breaking of addictions to coffee, tea, chocolate or alcohol will release the causes, which can then be explored, adjusted and transformed as a part of the healing process. The need for coffee may have its roots in exhaustion, liver malfunction, constipation or stress.

First, drinking other things leaves less space for drinking black tea and coffee, which deplete adrenal energy. After the initial stimulation, continued drinking accelerates the problem of exhaustion. If we are drinking four cups of herbal tea a day, that means four cups less black tea or coffee. The apple cider vinegar and honey drink eliminates another cup. Herbal nutrients support organs, systems and glands so that the root causes for caffeine addiction are relieved. As energy builds from within, the need for stimulation lessens, and soon patients find they enjoy coffee less and less and feel satisfied by herb teas, grain coffee, miso drinks and Dandelion root coffee.

If the underlying problem is lack of energy, exhaustion or fatigue after meals, then this is what needs to be treated. An iris analysis together with an in–depth case history will reveal the spectrum of habits and functional imbalances that cause exhaustion. After clients are educated about their unique body/emotion/mind/spirit dynamics, receive their individual program and put it into practice, the release from addictive indulgences and excesses becomes easier because it is supported by the rejuvenative processes within the body.

TAKE THESE FOODS OUT OF YOUR KITCHEN

Because one of the prime goals of purification and regeneration treatment is to eliminate excess toxins, acids and mucus from the body organs and tissues, it is essential that diet be adjusted, so that toxins are not being put back into the body as fast as they are being eliminated. The list below is a guide to the elimination of foods and drinks that contribute to the development of the chronic conditions that accompany aging and disease. Leave out the following foods and replace them with their substitutes. This will make a great contribution to our future health and quality of life.

ELIMINATE	SUBSTITUTE
Salt	Savory kitchen herbs, cayenne, ground dandelion greens, seaweeds, soy sauce
Tea, coffee, alcohol	Herbal teas, dandelion and grain coffees, warm juices, spices, miso drink, fresh juices; coffee and tea contain high levels of tannin that neutralizes iron; eliminate tea and coffee when taking herbal supplements
Sugar	Honey, maple syrup, dried fruits, fruit juices, other natural sweeteners, stevia, sweet root vegetables
Meat, fish, fowl, eggs	Tofu, nuts, seeds, high protein vegetables, Spirulina
Dairy products	A small amount of goat's milk products or soy cheese
Flour, pasta	Wheat flour is mucus–forming; use chickpea, millet, spelt, quinoa or rice flour; use whole grain, fresh, organic flour products only, without chemical additives and preservatives and processing
Soda, sugar sweetened drinks, carbonated drinks	Distilled water with a dash of lemon, herbal teas, fresh vegetable and fruit juices, miso drinks

One of the best approaches to the transition phase of the diet is to go through all the kitchen cupboards, pack away all of the foods to be eliminated and donate them to a homeless shelter. Then make up a shopping list of all of the recommended foods. When we only allow the foods that are good for us into our home, this makes it easier to eliminate other foods from our diets. Increase fresh fruit and vegetables, wholefood grains, nuts and seeds.

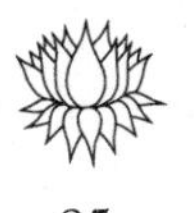

Add These Foods to Your Kitchen

Refer to the Nourishment charts in the Appendices that show acid and alkaline foods and the highest natural food and herb sources for all the vitamins and minerals. Eat sufficient amounts of fresh, organic premium foods to receive all the nourishment you need.

Alfalfa

This plant is an herbal, multi–vitamin, bowel cleanser and energy–giving food. Take two to four tablets or more per meal. The roots of the Alfalfa plant grow deeply into the earth where they seek out and draw up valuable trace elements and minerals. Alfalfa has a gently softening and laxative effect on the bowels.

Almond Milk

This is a tasty milk substitute for children and adults. Blanch one cup almonds then slip off the skins. Blend together with one quart water, one half teaspoon honey, and one tablespoon safflower oil. Strain the pulp and use it in soups, salads and casseroles.

Capsicum or Cayenne Pepper

Capsicum is a safe, pure stimulant, antiseptic and toning agent that helps the system throw off disease and establish equilibrium of circulation. Take one–quarter teaspoon in yogurt or tomato juice three times daily. Drink quickly and follow with a chaser. Increase the dose to one full teaspoon three times daily. Although it seems very hot and strong the taste buds soon adjust.

Honey and Apple Cider Vinegar

Mix one teaspoon honey and one tablespoon apple cider in one–quarter to one–half cup of warm water three times a day to soothe, balance and alkalinize the digestion. The high potassium and antiseptic qualities of this folk medicine drink have proven themselves over centuries.

Kelp

High mineral supplement and thyroid nutrient. Take six to twelve tablets daily.

Lecithin

The high phosphorus nutrient increases brain energy and reduces cholesterol levels.

Miso

Soybean miso provides alkalinizing, strengthening soup stocks and beverages that provide power, energy and warmth, and offer a healthy alternative to fruit or cereal breakfasts.

Potassium Broth

This broth provides nutritious, alkalinizing, pleasant, energy–giving meals. Soak two cups bran and one cup oatmeal overnight in one and one half quarts of water. Strain out the grain and keep the water. Add potatoes, carrots, onions, celery and parsley. Simmer gently in the bran–oatmeal water. Mash vegetables. Strain again to make broth. Season with herbs and Cayenne.

Seaweeds

Add seaweeds to soups and salads for their high mineral content. Macrobiotic books are an excellent guide to the use of seaweeds. Wash, tear and mix the raw seaweeds with salads or add to soups after they are cooked.

Spirulina

If hunger and cravings for sweet, sour or salty foods are a problem, bowel cleansing combined with a regular intake of Spirulina will help reduce cravings. When the cleansing current is most active, we need to support regeneration. Whereas other proteins stop the purification process, Spirulina balances purification with regeneration, so that both continue at a more comfortable level. One to three teaspoons of Spirulina per meal provides adequate protein. The addition of the Alkaline and Multi–Mineral and Vitamin formulae offers a full spectrum of nutritional supplementation.

Three Seeds

Powder a mixture of sunflower, sesame and pumpkin seeds and sprinkle over salads and vegetables for their high nutritive content.

Tofu

Soybean curd provides alkaline, easily digestible protein. As tofu has a bland, neutral flavor on its own, simmer lightly in soy sauce or tamari. Add fresh cut herbs, red, green or yellow peppers, green onions, Garlic, Ginger, and any other quick–cooking vegetable. Cut, dice and add to soups, stews and nut loaves. Use Turmeric or Saffron to color the tofu beautiful shades of golden yellow.

Wheat Germ Oil

One tablespoon of fresh oil will provide the vitamin E and other nutrients necessary to assist the healing process. Take in juice or on salads.

FASTING

I do not recommend fasting until the eliminative organs and systems are working at optimum levels and the alkaline purification diet has been followed for at least a month. Many people fast, deprive themselves, experience discomfort, and then feel they have accomplished something. However, unless the toxins are eliminated from the system, the fast is a waste of time and energy.

Prepare for a fast by going on a purification and rejuvenation program first. Once a level of balanced function is achieved and elimination is active, then consider a fast. Support the fast with baths, saunas, steambaths, enemas, colonics, reflexology, massage and exercise.

Plan a daily program. Write lists. Organize and shop for what will be needed during the fast. Take care of all errands and duties first. Choose good music and books. Enjoy nature. Allow time and space to rest, sleep, dream and heal. Create a nurturing atmosphere. My fasting experiences are some of my most beautiful memories. If the fast is done properly, it will be a special experience and a valuable contribution to your life.

Comfort Foods & Cravings

It is important not to be too strict or to deny ourselves foods we love or crave unless we are in a life–and–death chronic disease program. The tension and emotional imbalances caused by suppression of cravings and food desires accumulates and causes reactions, eventually resulting in binges, or reversal to negative eating patterns.

Food provides physical energy which goes downward through digestion, etheric energy which is absorbed through the palate to the central nervous system, emotional satisfaction which is calming, and delight to the senses, the eyes, nose, taste and touch. To deny any aspect of this range of nourishment is asking for trouble.

Over the years so many clients have said to me: "When I'm upset, I head for chocolate, bread and butter or toast and jam." Inability to express emotions or to complete a problem activates liver distress which is calmed by chewing, the smell of toast and the warm, soft, sweet comfort of carbohydrates. For others, the comfort is attained by chocolate, alcohol or coffee. We ultimately learn to see that the food that we crave is actually increasing the imbalance.

This craving is a very real need, and while some patients find the will and strength to stop indulging completely, others have a struggle. Strong cravings can be reduced by the use of Spirulina, six capsules, or a teaspoon mixed with juice one to three times a day. Acupuncture may also be needed to restore balance. Sometimes our jaw is tight because of emotions and shock, and the patient simply needs to chew. Sunflower seeds are excellent for this purpose.

Herbal treatment also eases cravings by providing superior nutrients for specific areas of need. As the body returns to balance, cravings diminish. Diets should not be made so rigid and strict that other imbalances or reactions occur. Because the herbal nutrients are so effective we can avoid strict diets, especially in the early stages of treatment. The elimination of harmful foods should be a comfortable natural process which happens gradually. As strength and balance are created from within, a wholesome diet becomes easier and easier to maintain. Slowly, the enjoyment for vital, natural foods returns, and the cravings for stimulants or synthetic tastes diminish or cease altogether.

It takes time for the tongue's taste buds to return to balance. If we have experienced cravings for any taste, whether sweet, sour, salty, bitter or pungent, this reflects elemental, emotional, chakra and meridian imbalances. One of the ways to adjust and balance the taste is to eat foods once a day which contain all the tastes. For instance, in the morning eat oatmeal garnished with the five tastes provided by honey, salt, horseradish, Ginger and chutney. When we take herb powders in juice, water or liquid yogurt, the bitter taste of the herbs will also help to heal the taste buds on the tongue.

Years ago when I first went to England, I could not enjoy the food, which was made with strong and excessive sugar, salt and spicy seasonings. I had been eating raw food for two years and had grown to love the pure taste of natural foods garnished with lemon juice, soy sauce and fresh herbs.

Do not assume that correct eating will not be enjoyable and satisfying. The taste buds rejoice in vital, fresh, simpler foods which leave us with a feeling of well–being. When we want to occasionally enjoy food for pure pleasure, our body will be able to handle it. We will be in control, no longer at the mercy of blind cravings or habits which are potentially destructive to our good health.

Purification Diet

This diet will help the return to normal weight. We will receive more vitality and satisfaction from food, cleanse our system and save considerably on our food budget. Do not be concerned that this diet omits meat and dairy proteins. Remember that cows, horses, elephants and even gorillas eat only plants, grains, nuts and seeds. Human beings thrive on vegetarian diets that are balanced and part of a healthy life style.

On Waking: Bach flower remedy; herbal tea or lemon and maple syrup in hot water; wait at least fifteen minutes before eating

Breakfast: Liver cleanse drink and wait one half an hour

Take herbal nutrients and supplements, immediately before a breakfast of low–cooked whole–grain cereal; fruit or a miso drink

At night, fill one third of a thermos with whole grain organic cereal; fill with boiling water; shake a few times and let it sit overnight; in the morning the grain should be soft; add olive oil and honey; low–heat cooking preserves the full nutrition and the cereal is still a live food

Mid–morning: Herb teas; fresh juice; Bach flower remedy

Lunch: Tossed salad of mixed vegetables, leafy greens, fresh cut herbs together with an oil and apple cider vinegar dressing, and a dash of lemon juice; use Garlic; add 8 to 10 blanched almonds and seaweeds; sprinkle the salad with the three–seed powder and lecithin, and take with regular herbal medicines and supplements; if lunch is the main meal of the day, add steamed or baked vegetables, potassium broth, soups or baked potatoes, sweet potatoes or yams; season potatoes with a tasty mixture of soy sauce, olive oil and Cayenne pepper

Afternoon: Bach flower remedy

Drink fresh juices during the afternoon; alternate carrot, grape, apple or vegetable mixtures; if bottled juices are necessary be sure to choose brands which are sugarless and free of preservatives

Evening meals: If the lunch was light, take a heavier meal at night; if lunch was the main meal, eat fruit salad with seeds, nuts, goat's yogurt, honey and soaked dried fruit; if sugar levels need to be reduced, prepare vegetable or miso soup instead

Before bed: Juices; warm beverages; fruit; Bach flower remedy; herbs as needed

Purifying Juice Cleanse

This juice cleanse will eliminate toxic lymph, mucus, catarrh and excess acids. It will help to normalize the weight and prepare the body for regeneration. This cleanse provides the highest nutritive and vibratory foods to rebuild vital parts of the body, eliminates frustration and confusion, raises cell regeneration above cell destruction, and expels negativity.

After rising in the morning, drink a half glass of prune juice. This draws toxins and eliminates them through the bowels as well as relieving constipation.

In the morning make two quarts of fresh juice, or buy the best quality organic juice in glass containers without sugar or preservatives. Mix this with two quarts of distilled water or with the best low mineral content spring water available in glass bottles. One half hour after drinking the prune juice, drink an eight ounce glass of the chosen juice and water mixture.

Every half hour throughout the day drink a glass of the diluted juice. If hungry, eat the fruit or vegetable of the chosen juice in the evening. For example, if it is an apple juice cleanse, eat an apple in the evening. If hunger is a problem, mix a spoon of Spirulina into the juice.

Every day take two tablespoons of cold–pressed olive oil to lubricate the liver and bile ducts. Small amounts in juice during the day will provide the required dose. The three–day cleanse can be repeated several times by alternating a different juice for the next three–day period. It is also wise to alternate between fruit which is cleansing, and vegetables which are regenerating, so that balance is maintained. A coffee enema or herbal enema mix will relieve cleansing headaches, aches and pains, especially if taken first thing in the morning and last thing at night.. Take prune juice if needed. Make sure the bowels are active. Take the herbal nutrient mix as usual during the day. If you are not on an herbal program, take the Bowel Rejuvenator formula on its own, two capsules per meal and adjust dosage as required.

After one or more of the three–day cycles, it is essential to break the cleanse properly. Start with a fruit salad for breakfast. Add honey and finely grated blanched almonds on top. Drink one or two glasses of fruit or vegetable juice in the morning. For lunch eat another fruit salad and drink vegetable juice during the afternoon. For the evening meal take a full vegetable salad with a simple salad dressing of pure cold pressed olive oil, apple cider vinegar, lemon and fresh cut culinary herbs.

When conditions are ideal it is beneficial to fast one to three days on water at the end of the juice cleanse. However, when breaking the water fast, first have one day on the juice cleanse before eating fruit and vegetable salads. Do not eat any heavy foods immediately. Add them gradually to your diet. Take an enema each morning of the water fast, and more often if needed.

Most people tell us they experience an increase in energy and a feeling of light well–being. Friends tell them their eyes are shining and that their skin glows. A properly conducted cleanse will not be a suffering experience if you adjust reactions with rest, enemas, aromatherapy, baths, exercise, fresh air, breathing, releasing emotion, and meditation.

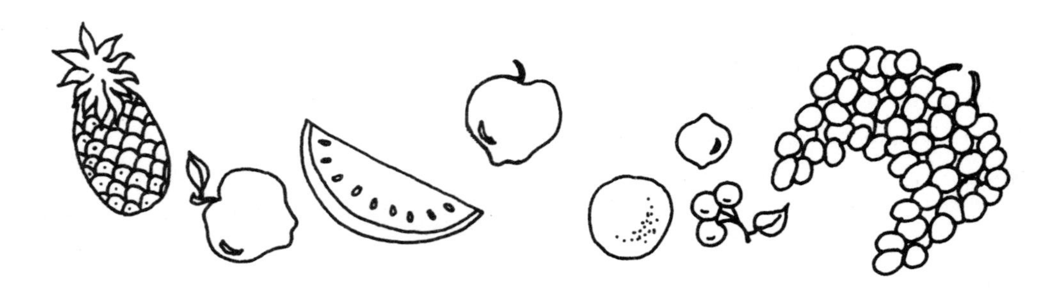

Mono Diet

This simple but powerful diet provides the digestive system with a rest almost as complete as a water or juice fast, together with the comfort, warmth, energy and strength that comes from eating foods which you enjoy and digest well. This is especially important if it is necessary to work full time, take care of a family or fast during physical, emotional or mental trauma, or during winter. Because the body is relieved from having to digest complicated combinations of food, it is able to focus on healing.

Whenever there are strong digestive symptoms such as a swollen abdomen, digestive cramps or pain, hiatus hernia or extreme gas, and it is not possible to do a water or juice fast, the mono diet gives superb results within one month. Support the mono diet with the full holistic regimen, including Bach flower remedies, naturopathic home treatments and herbal formulae.

Choose one food at a time for each meal – a fruit, vegetable or a grain. Eat as much of that food as you like. Take a meal as often as required, several times a day if desired, as long as they are at least one hour apart, to allow time to completely digest each food.

Use only cold pressed oils, lemon or cider vinegar, or Cayenne pepper to improve the flavor and assist digestion. Foods can be taken raw, steamed or baked depending on the season, individual energy requirements, what digests most easily and individual preferences.

As the month progresses it becomes clear which foods digest well and which foods cause reactions. Foods which cause any discomfort should be eliminated from the diet. After taking each food note the results, whether you feel light or heavy, alert or sleepy, satisfied or still hungry.

Choose a variety of foods. Include all foods within the suggested whole food, vegetarian, alkaline guidelines. When it is time to return to a more normal diet, the foods which caused aggravations should be eliminated from the diet for at least three months. When they are reintroduced watch carefully for any reactions.

Drink fresh juices from one fruit or vegetable at a time, herb teas, lemon with apple cider vinegar and honey and pure distilled water. These can be taken cool or warm, but not hot or cold.

Herbal supplements can be taken with the meals. If there are a number of meals throughout the day reduce the dose per meal, so that herbs are taken with each meal.

Although it may be difficult to imagine how satisfying a meal of steamed beets or baked squash can be, make a start and let experience demonstrate the benefits of this healing diet.

Often when there has been a shock, due to death, loss or accident, the digestive system malfunctions. This diet will help the digestive system return to normal without causing a strain. It is important to eat light, satisfying foods which are pleasantly presented during stressful times.

Tasty & Healthy Energy Snacks

If the metabolism is overactive and food moves quickly through the digestive system, or the expenditure of energy is considerable, loss of weight or hunger may occur on purifying or health–building diets. Also, large or tall persons, or those who are active over long hours or do physical work, require more food to sustain them. It is important to take regular snacks during the day to provide the required nourishment. However, do not eat continuously, as this will not allow proper digestion of each meal or snack. The following suggestions will help expand the diet program.

Mix dried fruit, seed and nut mixes. Keep a bag of raisins, currants, dates, nuts and seeds nearby for regular snacks, or for when hunger strikes. Spirulina bars are very nutritious for snacks.

Add extra Multi–Vitamin Mineral formula to the herbal nutrients. Take higher doses of herbs, more often, to reduce hunger and increase energy and strength.

Miso soup or Spirulina drinks contribute a potent balancing and nourishing effect which reduce the need for sweets or stimulants that provide immediate energy but leave you depleted.

If the metabolism is hyperactive through nervous or glandular imbalance, it may be necessary to add extra herbs to soothe, calm and slow down body functions. The problem could also be associated with a malfunctioning ileo–caecal valve (which determines when food is to be released from the small intestine into the large intestine), constipation, stress, excessive emotions or anxiety. The Exhaustion formula or Gentian root will increase the body's ability to absorb nutrients.

Longitudinal ridges on the nails indicate diminished ability to absorb nutrients. As the digestion improves the nails will grow normally again.

Acid/Alkaline Balance

Science has divided foods, like chemicals, into two classes: alkaline–forming or positive, safe foods and acid–forming or negative, unhealthy ones. If we eat over 80% alkaline foods this helps to preserve the normal alkalinity of the blood. This is an important key to balancing foods. Although some items are acid forming, do not exclude them entirely. Use them judiciously, and in the correct balance, so they will yield the greatest good.

Rest and sleep are alkalizers. So are exercise, fresh air, pleasure, laughter, good conversation, enjoyment – especially love! Complete hot baths and showers with cool or cold showers for an alkalinizing and energizing effect. Try it! Feel more awake and alive. Acidifiers are worry, fear, anger, gossip, hatred, envy, selfishness and greed, so cleanse these out of the system as well.

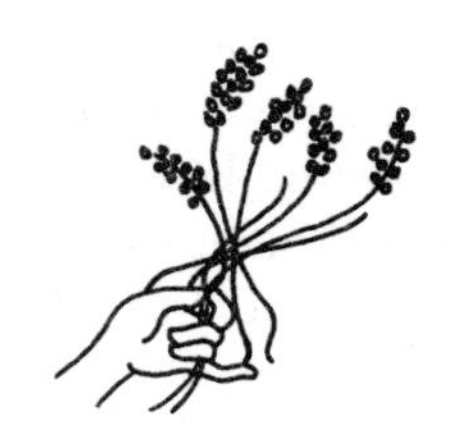

Liver Cleanse Drink For a Purifying Diet

Dr. Randolph Stone, the originator of polarity therapy, recommends a cold pressed organic olive oil mixed with lemon as a liver cleanser and healer. Cooked and fried oils create stress for the liver. During healing programs avoid all cooked and fried oils. Take the liver cleanse drink daily to support the herbal nutrients, dietary changes and home treatments, and to rejuvenate the liver. Do not use the drink on a daily basis for longer than a month. Take a break for a couple of weeks and then use it again.

Daily breakfast: mix three to four tablespoons pure cold pressed, organic almond, olive or sesame seed oil in six to eight tablespoons (twice the oil amount) of fresh squeezed lemon juice. Add fresh Ginger juice and grapefruit, orange or tangerine juice to taste. Blend with three to six cloves of Garlic. Drink and follow with a herbal tea containing Licorice, Anise, Fennel, and Fenugreek (simmered together on a very low heat) then add Peppermint and Violet leaves. Infuse until the mixture is cool enough to drink. Chew the citrus seeds in the mouth for fifteen minutes to gain the benefit of enzymes, vitamins and minerals. The bitter essence is helpful to the liver and also helps relieve any Garlic odor especially when used along with Parsley or whole Cloves. Do not take food with this cleanse drink.

Constipation: add higher amounts of Licorice root and fresh Garlic.

Diarrhea: do not use Licorice, Ginger or the liver cleanse drink. Substitute Cinnamon bark tea, or use ground Cinnamon generously mixed with baked or cooked apples or cooked with rice or barley. Mullein tea is a specific herb for diarrhea.

Castor Oil Pack: support the liver cleanse drink with a Castor oil pack over the liver area three days a week. Refer to the pack instructions in the Herbal and Naturopathy Treatments chapter.

Reflexology: massage the liver and gall bladder reflex areas on the feet to support the effect of the liver cleanse drink. Have a polarity therapy or reflexology treatment once or twice a week.

Liver Cleanse Drink for a Rejuvenating Diet

Take one to three tablespoons of pure cold–pressed almond or olive oil mixed with three times the amount of fresh lime or lemon juice followed by two cups of hot water with the juice of one half of one lime or lemon juice to each cupful. Alternately take one eight ounce glass of fresh orange, grapefruit, pineapple or pomegranate juice with one–third tablespoon of cold pressed oil, followed by two cups of hot lemon water. This also helps to relieve constipation.

The rejuvenating liver cleanse drink may be followed by fresh fruit with a few almonds and raisins about fifteen minutes later. A heavier breakfast may be taken one hour later.

Use three–quarters of a cup of millet and one–quarter cup Fenugreek to make steamed porridge in a thermos overnight. Add fresh pressed Ginger juice to one cup water in which raisins, dates or figs were soaked overnight, and mix with the steamed grains.

Total Nourishment

Nourishment is also reflected in other aspects of life. Add satisfying activities that will increase the ability to receive true and healthy nourishment. We need to learn how to take care of ourselves, enjoy doing the things that will make us feel good, and bring happiness and well–being into our lives.

Exercise

Movement is life! Exercise is essential. Whether we choose vigorous walking, jogging, aerobics, dancing, swimming, yoga, tai chi, home bouncers or gym workouts, it is necessary to stimulate circulation, exercise muscles, stretch, tone and activate the lymphatic system.

Breathing

Deep breathing is essential to bring in life–giving oxygen and to eliminate poisonous gases and toxins. If there is difficulty in breathing fully for five minutes twice a day, take up yoga, tai chi and low impact aerobic workouts. Just walking up a gentle slope will deepen the breath. Expand the chest by holding the hands behind while you walk, like the Sherpa trek porters do in the Himalayas.

Vital Circuitry

Walk barefoot for at least fifteen minutes per day to ground the accumulation of static electricity and release stagnant energy. Wear cotton or natural fiber socks and comfortable natural shoes, or open sandals to allow the feet to relax. Walk barefoot around home whenever possible. Disciplines such as tai chi and dance utilize sensitive foot movements which revive and awaken the feet, benefiting the entire being. Have a weekly reflexology treatment to restore circulation and energy to the feet.

Natural Fibers

Synthetic fabrics build up static electricity around the body and inhibit skin function. Wear only cotton, silk, linen and wool cloth and make sure all bedding is 100% cotton. Use quilts made from natural feathers and down, never synthetic fillers. Health is more important than easy laundry care. Never use electric blankets because they reduce the body's ability to produce its own body heat. Short–term comfort is paid for by long–term imbalances in the natural healing functions of the body, not to mention the effect the electricity has on the body's vital circuitry.

Mental and Spiritual Attitudes

Think positively. Know that it is possible to be healthy. Be grateful for this opportunity for healing. Be willing to release toxins and the mental and emotional patterns that created them, and like the phoenix become renewed. Live from the growing edge. Cooperate abundantly with life as it unfolds. Old outer layers will die away and leave room for the new self to emerge. Imagine being at the center of an expanding flower and feel the beauty of that growth. Practice visualizations and positive thinking. Study and practice meditation regularly.

6

Herbal & Naturopathy Treatments

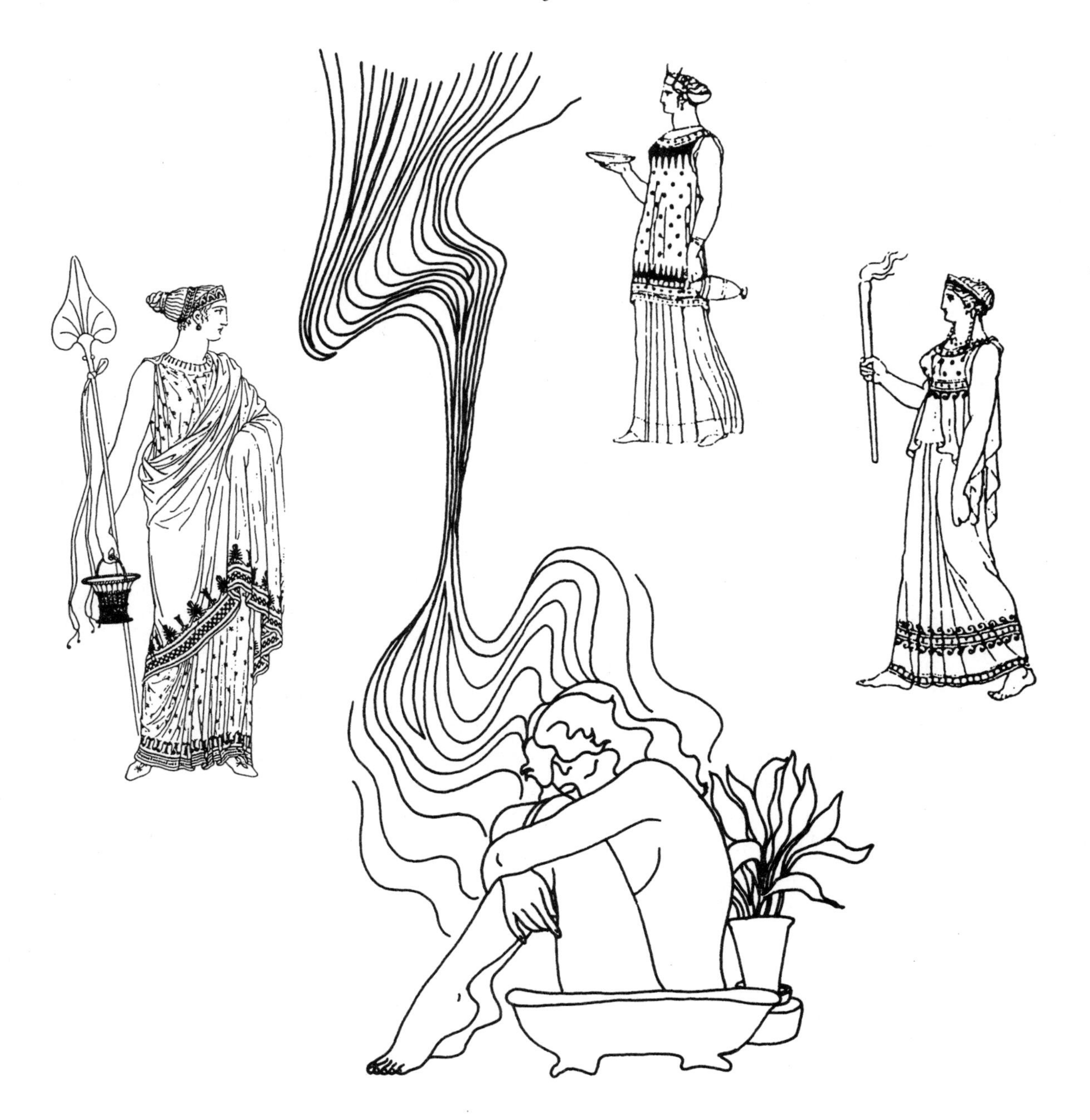

Herbal and Naturopathy Treatments

This chapter gives detailed information for the uses of self–help home treatments that support the herbal nutrients, and the purifying and rejuvenative diets. Results are augmented and accelerated when these treatments are used.

The treatments are simple and inexpensive. They can be worked into a busy life in the evenings and weekend leisure hours, while watching television or reading books, and during sleep. They can also be used for preventive, maintenance, acute or chronic care.

The results of these treatments prove that simple naturopathy treatments in combination with herbs relieve pain, detoxify specific and systemic congestion, activate circulation, increase elimination, and achieve relaxation. Try these treatments and experience their benefits so that you are familiar with them and can apply them easily and quickly during times of need.

Abdominal Packs

Cold Abdominal Pack

Buy two cloths, one of 100% firmly woven cotton and the other of 100% pliable wool, to make two wraps exactly the same, each 18" wide x 60" long. The eighteen inches width of the cloth will fit from under the ribs to the top of the thighs, covering the full abdomen. The sixty inches length is wrapped around the body, making three or more layers depending on the person's size. A small person, a child or a very large person may require a cloth made to size. Ultimately there should be a minimum of three thicknesses of each of the cotton and wool cloths. The cotton cloth moisturizes and the wool cloth increases the temperature because it helps to hold in the body heat.

Wet the cotton cloth in cold water, wring out and wrap quickly around your body twice, covering the torso from the groin to the bottom of the ribs. This will feel cold and uncomfortable for just a moment, but as soon as the wool is wrapped around the body heat will immediately warm the pack. Once the wool top cloth is secure, tie the entire pack into place with a thick cotton ribbon or string, wear a body stocking which holds it in place, or use stretch bandages to wrap around the waist.

The best time to apply the pack is in the evening at least two hours after eating. It is necessary to wear it for an hour and a half, but it can also be removed in the morning. When it is removed it is usually still damp. It is perfectly alright to walk around, sit up or lie down.

The abdominal pack increases circulation, activates metabolic functions, stimulates kidney activity, reduces inflammation and calms the nervous system. It produces a feeling of well–being and relief if there is pain or congestion in digestive, reproductive or urinary organs. In case of vomiting and nausea the cold abdominal pack relieves the pancreas and slows down and eventually stops the vomiting. The pack also tones and tightens the abdominal muscles.

Constipation must be relieved completely for this treatment to work effectively. Use enemas, Castor oil packs and herbal supplements to activate and cleanse the bowels.

Mud Pack

Mud packs reduce intestinal inflammation when applied twice a day over a period of time. These are made with natural earth that has never been sprayed with insecticide or fertilized with chemicals. Sift and strain the earth until it is a fine consistency, and then mix with water to form a thick mud. Shape the pack by spreading two inches of the mud over a thick 100% cotton cloth that has been placed over the entire bottom and sides of a wood box the size of your abdomen. Let the mud set until it is firm. Lift the pack out by pulling the cloth, then turn it so that the mud is placed directly on the abdominal skin. Cover with a towel and rest with the pack on for twenty minutes to one–half hour. Make a small mud pack to cool and freshen the eyes at the same time. The mud draws out toxins, tones the muscles and cools and reduces inflammation.

Although these abdominal packs seem like simple treatments, the effects are powerful. Don't underestimate their influence on internal organs and systems. They are especially helpful to increase circulation to the kidneys. Use nightly during any fasting and purification program. Whenever I fast at the Institute of Naturopathic and Yogic Sciences in India, I receive two mud packs a day, one in the morning at 8 a.m. and one at about 1 p.m. The cold abdominal pack is also given every evening. These treatments augment the cleansing, rejuvenating and healing effects of the fast.

Acute Illnesses & Accidents

Whenever illnesses occur, consider how your lifestyle has produced the condition. Has there been a change of diet or location? Is there exhaustion, insomnia, stress, anxiety, emotional excess or shock? Illness is usually the result of disordered living. Even accidents are the result of confusion, disorientation, absent–mindedness or karmic retribution. The condition and where the wound is often reveal information about the issues that have come to the surface in a dramatic way. Do not resort to allopathic or suppressive measures unless there is a life and death emergency. Take heart. Have the courage to weather the illness and support the body's work to heal the acute condition. Stop eating a regular diet. Choose any of the following diets: water fast, juice cleanse, purifying diet or mono diet. Drink cleansing herbal teas, such as Pau D'Arco.

Bruises

Use homeopathic *Arnica* internally and externally, together with hot and cold water applications, poultices, and the Bach flower *Rescue Remedy*.

Burns

Bach flower *Rescue Remedy*, homeopathic *Cantharis*, cold water, Aloe Vera gel, homeopathic burn ointment and the burn and wound paste in this chapter.

Cramps

Administer the Calcium, Nerve and Adrenal herbal formulae internally in acute doses, together with soothing aromatherapy and Epsom salts baths and homeopathic *Colocynthis*.

Diarrhea

Administer homeopathic *Veratrum*, *Chinchona* or *Ipecacuanha*, and Mullein infusion.

Fever, Colds & Flu Treatment

Work with a fever. Recognize the good work it is attempting to do. Take a hot bath which contains a tablespoon each of Ginger powder, Cayenne powder and Mustard powder. Cleanse the colon with enemas before the bath. Make the bath as hot as possible, and soak for at least one half hour. Cold cloths on the head and neck will help to balance the heat. Drink hot Yarrow or Peppermint tea in the bath. Sponge down with apple cider vinegar, and then climb immediately into bed. Cover up with quilts and blankets with hot water bottles at the feet and around the body. Stay in bed at least until normal body temperature is restored.

Whenever there are extreme fevers, wrap up first in a wet sheet before covering up with the quilts and hot water bottles. The wet sheet causes a stronger reaction and draws out more toxins. Stay in bed at least two hours (or until the body cools naturally) to allow full perspiration to take place. Continue drinking Yarrow or Peppermint tea. Get up, shower, dress in cotton pajamas, walk about, breathe fresh air, go outside if possible, and then return to bed for further rest. If these therapies are followed the illness will be of short duration, and the body will return to normal more quickly, with the added benefits of cleansing, rest and the elimination of toxins.

Flower Remedies

Support any imbalance in emotions and mental attitudes with flower remedies. Once feelings and thoughts have eased, physical healing can take place much more quickly and easily. The Bach flower *Rescue Remedy* mix should be administered as quickly as possible to prevent complications from accidents, injuries, shock or trauma and to relieve shock and confusion by opening up life energies for healing. Take four drops every five to ten minutes on the tongue. Rub it on the head and body. Take a bath with two dropperfulls of the remedy in the water.

Dosage for acute conditions: take four drops on the tongue, or in a small amount of water every fifteen minutes or more often. Do not touch the dropper to the tongue. During accidents and traumas take four drops every five minutes, decreasing the doses in five minute increments until the doses are one–half hour apart. When recovery is progressing take every hour. Complete the treatment with four drops of *Rescue Remedy* four times a day until the condition has cleared and the mind and emotions have recovered their balance.

Dosage for long–term conditions of any remedy mixture: take four drops hourly during waking hours for three to five days whenever you are dedicated to a purification, rejuvenation and transformation program. Then adjust to the regular dose of four times daily. Remember, it is important to take the first dose on waking and the last just before going to sleep. Put it on the kitchen sink during the day when at home. It is convenient to have two bottles of the remedy: one in a purse or pocket for travelling or work, and one at home.

Heart Attacks & Strokes

Immediately give a teaspoon of Cayenne in tomato juice or warm water, and repeat every five or ten minutes. Put the person in a Cayenne, and Lobelia bath to equalize and balance blood flow. Call for medical help. Supplement the diet with appropriate herbal teas and herbal formulae. Use herbs with the treatments as directed.

Hemorrhages

Immediately drink several teaspoons of Cayenne dissolved in tomato or pineapple juice, or warm water, and put large amounts on the wound or source of hemorrhage, such as the vagina after giving birth. This equalizes the circulation and draws blood from the area. Homeopathic *Phosphorus* will also help. Do not be concerned about the hot taste of the Cayenne when life is in danger from loss of blood. This treatment could save lives while waiting for medical assistance.

Inflammation

Alternating hot and cold water baths or applications reduce inflammation and increase healing because the heat draws the blood and the cold sends it away, increasing circulation. Do this as quickly as possible after any sprain or break to avoid swelling and inflammation.

Insect bites

Immediately use *Rescue Remedy* and homeopathic *Ledum* and *Apis*. Pack clay or mud on the bite to draw out the poison. Go to emergency for extremely poisonous bites. Use Mullein and Slippery Elm poultices.

Lightning Strikes

Once my daughter, Casel, was injured by lightning in the Rocky Mountains. Luckily I was near, and even though she was in convulsions she did not pass out. Because she did not have burns on her hands and feet, I knew it was not a direct hit. For the first half hour I rubbed her face and body with Rescue Remedy and kept putting the drops in her mouth. After each dose the convulsions calmed. When she was able to move, I carried her over to the kitchen sink and helped her hold on to the metal pipes, so the excess electric charge could drain out of her body. This worked wonders. The next step was a long soak in an aromatherapy bath. An hour and a half after the lightning strike she was sitting up watching a video and drinking cocoa. We called it her enlightening experience!

Rashes & Itching

Wrap or place cloths soaked in Chickweed over the affected area, or take a Chickweed bath. The Allergy and the Lymphatic formulae will help the immune system to overcome the condition. Homeopathic *Arsenicum* or *Rhus Tox* are useful, as are *Rescue Remedy* baths.

Tooth pain

Homeopathic *Hypericum* relieves nerve pain. Rub Clove oil on the teeth and gums. Take White Willow bark herb internally in either powder or tincture form to relieve pain. Use alternating hot and cold poultices over the painful area. Press the reflexology tooth areas on the toes and finger,s and massage the jaw muscles and neck glands.

Vomiting

Drink salt water and cleanse the stomach. Take Peppermint tea. Use a cold abdominal Pack. Rub the reflexology stomach points on the feet. Take homeopathic *Ipecacuanha*.

The above is a short list to give ideas and approaches for acute treatment. There are many wonderful reference works – herbal, homeopathic and naturopathic – that contain a full range of information to guide and assist treatment for acute situations. When you experience the help that these simple and basic remedies and treatments give, explore further, extend the range of information, and build a reference library.

Bath Therapies

Choose a quiet time for a daily bath. This is a time for rest and rejuvenation, so set the stage with love. Light candles and incense, bring in music or a book, or float away and forget the world with visualizations, dreams or meditation.

Pour the bath as hot as possible. If there are heart problems or high blood pressure, adjust the temperature to suit the condition. While the water is running, scrub and brush the skin with loofahs, mitts or natural bristle brushes. Brush in circular motions moving away from the periphery of the body towards the center of the body and the heart.

At least once a week, remove dead skin by rubbing the body with Epsom salts. This leaves the skin feeling soft and clean and enables the skin to function fully.

Aromatherapy Baths

The addition of aromatherapy oils can help achieve relaxation, uplift the spirits and stimulate the various lymphatic glands, body systems and organs. They also provide a fragrant, lovely bath experience. Buy a book and invest in a selection of oils. My favorite oils are:

Fragrance	*Attribute*
Chamomile	Relaxing
Sandalwood	Uplifting
Juniper	Diuretic
Lavender	Aches and Pains
Rosemary	Fatigue

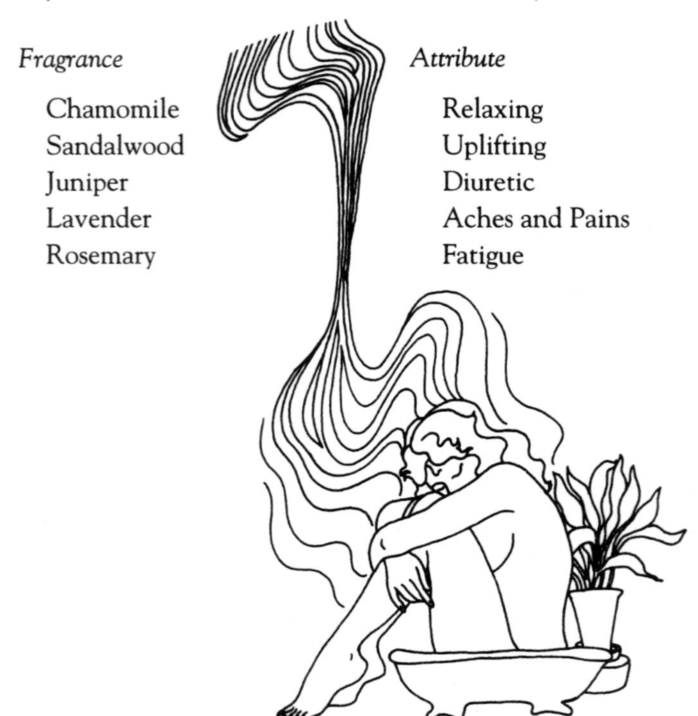

Epsom Salts/Cider Vinegar Baths

Mix four tablespoons of almond or olive oil into one or more cups of commercial Epsom salts, (not the finely ground, expensive internal brand), and then rub the mixture all over the body while standing in the bathtub. This removes old skin, leaving it smooth and soft, and the salts fall into the bathtub. Pour the bath as hot as possible, add one cup apple cider vinegar and stir. Soak for at least one half hour. Keep adding hot water. Place a cold cloth on the forehead and on the back of the neck. This bath is relaxing, and reduces aches, pain and fatigue after exercise and when on purification programs. Epsom salts draw out toxins and feed the body with magnesium.

Complete this bath with a cool spray, then wrap up in quilts so that the body perspires freely. It is also helpful to drink cupfuls of stimulating teas to encourage free perspiration from the skin. While Yarrow tea is the strongest, Sage, Catnip, Pleurisy root, Peppermint or Spearmint are also effective.

Saunas and Turkish Baths

Today there are many sauna and steam facilities available in hotels, health clubs and massage and treatment centers. In the winter they are effective for eliminating toxins, stimulating the circulation and relieving tense muscles caused by contracting against the cold weather. Scrub your skin during the sauna and make sure you take cold showers to balance the heat expansion, send the blood back to the interior of your body, close the pores and alkalinize the blood. Dry your hair thoroughly and dress warmly before going outside. It is good to walk and breathe deeply to complete this rejuvenative treatment.

Herbal Baths

Lobelia	Very relaxing, gives an excellent sleep
Catnip	Relaxing and soothing, excellent for children
Chamomile	Gently relaxing, uplifts the spirit
Capsicum, Ginger and Mustard	Stimulating, warming; equalizes circulation to the extremities; overcomes chills, colds and flu
Chaparral	Purifying; supports elimination

If you have had a very hot bath it is necessary to complete the bath by cooling the skin, closing the pores and balancing hot with cold. Pour cold water into the bath while the hot is running out. Take a cold or cool shower, splash yourself all over with cold water, and walk around naked for at least fifteen minutes. Sunbathe nude, either inside with the window open, or outside if the weather is warm. If you wish to produce copious perspiration to eliminate the onset of a chill, cold or flu, go directly from the hot bath to a very warm bed packed with hot water bottles, or exercise actively to produce full perspiration, until the body cools down naturally.

Hand and Foot Baths

Healing proceeds rapidly when hands and feet are soaked in strong herbal infusions and decoctions. Absorption into the capillaries in the extremities allows full absorption of the nutrients directly in the blood and lymph, thus feeding the body much more quickly than through digestion. Very useful for leg ulcers, swollen ankles, kidney afflictions, blood poisoning and healing specific areas.

Hip Baths

Cold hip baths are effective to reduce uterine bleeding and decrease pelvic inflammation. The cold sends the blood away from the surface of the skin and reduces congestion. Three minutes twice a day will produce an excellent effect when combined with dietary, herbal and naturopathic therapies. Mud packs can also be applied twice daily over the abdomen to support this treatment.

Sitz Baths

Cold sitz baths increase circulation to the pelvis area and activate nerve stimulation. Sit in a bowl or a small tub of cold water with the legs out, so that only the genitals and lower pelvis are submerged. Start with one minute at a time, but sit no longer than three minutes. Do not dry or rub with towels. Put on cotton pajamas and walk briskly after the sitz bath.

Alternating hot and cold sitz baths are very effective when treating reproductive conditions such as uterine fibroid tumors and vaginitis. Always end with a cold application. Apply this treatment only once or twice a day.

Hot sitz baths, taken from three to eight minutes at a time, twice a day, are useful for sub–acute conditions such as inflammation of the fallopian tubes.

Sprays

The use of alternate hot and cold sprays on areas of arthritis, stiffness, stroke or injury increases the flow of circulation, especially when the person is not able to exercise. During this treatment the blood is alkalinized and healing processes are stimulated. These sprays are also helpful for treating reproductive diseases since stagnant blood and poor circulation are often contributing factors. Use a hose while the person is standing or sitting. Water temperatures should be as hot and as cold as possible without causing undue discomfort. Allow three to five minutes for each spray before changing and repeat several times. Dress in cotton clothes and walk briskly after the treatment.

Bath & Body Products

Choose only natural bath and body oils and lotions. Make sure the body is not exposed to any product that could not be considered food because the body absorbs all substances put on the skin and must assimilate or eliminate them through its body purification systems. Mix a base of almond oil with smaller amounts of coconut, jojoba and avocado oils for a beautiful and healthy body lotion. Add an aromatherapy oil for fragrance and specific benefits you may want, such as help with cellulite, fatigue, or aches and pains. After pumicing old skin or calluses, rub the feet thoroughly with natural oils.

Castor oil is also a valuable beauty product. It moisturizes the deepest layers of the skin and leaves the skin soft and supple. Rub the oil on the face and then steam with two or three hot cloths. Complete the treatment with a cool or cold cloth or dip the face in a cold bowl of water for as long as you can. This will increase circulation and tighten and tone the facial muscles.

Burn and Wound Paste

Liquidize equal parts of honey, wheat germ or vitamin E oil, and finely ground and sifted Comfrey herb powder. Apply a spreadable paste one half inch thick over the burned area. Cover with gauze and a stretch bandage, to hold in place. Use a thinner mixture in any area where there is constant active body movement. Moisten the paste with a thin mixture of the above as the body heat dries out the poultice. Never allow any rough pieces in the poultice mix. Sift the herb powder if necessary because rough pieces will irritate the wound. Burn poultices must be left on and continuously replenished by either pure water or moist applications of fresh poultice.

On no account remove the poultice until the skin is completely healed and the poultice falls off by itself. This may take three weeks or longer. If it has to come off because it gets too dry, or it begins to smell, follow directions in the next paragraph.

Never pull the poultice off. It must be gently soaked in an herbal antibiotic bath of Thyme, Tea Tree, Golden Seal and Echinacea. Seek professional guidance because individual decisions must be made daily in dealing with all the reactions of the patient. The poultice is rebuilding skin, and must not be disturbed.

Burn poultices should be supported by the use of internal herbal nutrients such as the Antibiotics Naturally, Lymphatic and Multi–Vitamin/Mineral formulae to provide all the nutrient necessary to support the healing process. It is useful to take vitamin E internally during the healing process. The poultice must be maintained immaculately. This treatment is not to be done in a casual way. It is also important to rest and move gently and not to disturb the poultice.

Healing severe burns takes several weeks, and the process must be monitored daily and great care taken. When done properly, this treatment results in complete healing, without scars or chelated tissue and without the infections, pain and scraping of more orthodox medical treatment. A scab forms over the burn which is continuously fed with the formulae. This rebuilds the skin tissue, and when it falls off fresh pink skin is revealed.

Keep burns out of direct sunlight for over a year after the healing. It is necessary to cover the area whenever it is exposed to the sun or the skin may be damaged.

Candida & Yeast Infections

French aromatherapists have made great strides in the use of aromatherapy oils in the vagina to reduce the yeast and bacterial infections which cause so much discomfort and distress to women. Thyme or Tea Tree oil are the most effective and can be used safely as needed over a long period of time. Use as a part of the ovule treatment, or alone.

Vaginal Douche

Inject, and retain inside the vagina for at least five minutes, one cup of strained herbal tea. Use a second cup as a douche. Yellow Dock, Echinacea, Tea Tree or Chickweed herbal infusions also make excellent douches, as does pure wheatgrass juice.

Vaginal Ovule

Thyme and Tea Tree oil can also be incorporated directly into the ovules. Disperse three drops of Tea Tree oil in a teaspoon of warm coconut oil and mix with the herbal powders. Roll into ovule shapes, then cut into one–inch lengths. Follow the treatment schedule as outlined in the full vaginal ovule treatment information at the end of this chapter.

When treating Candida Albicans it is essential to follow a yeast–free diet, eliminate most acid forming foods and reach a level of full eliminative function. The harmonious balance of organs and systems within the full spectrum of spiritual/mental/emotional/physical health is also essential. It is recommended that any treatment for Candida be accompanied by a full constitutional herbal treatment based on an iridology analysis, and by a complete change in diet.

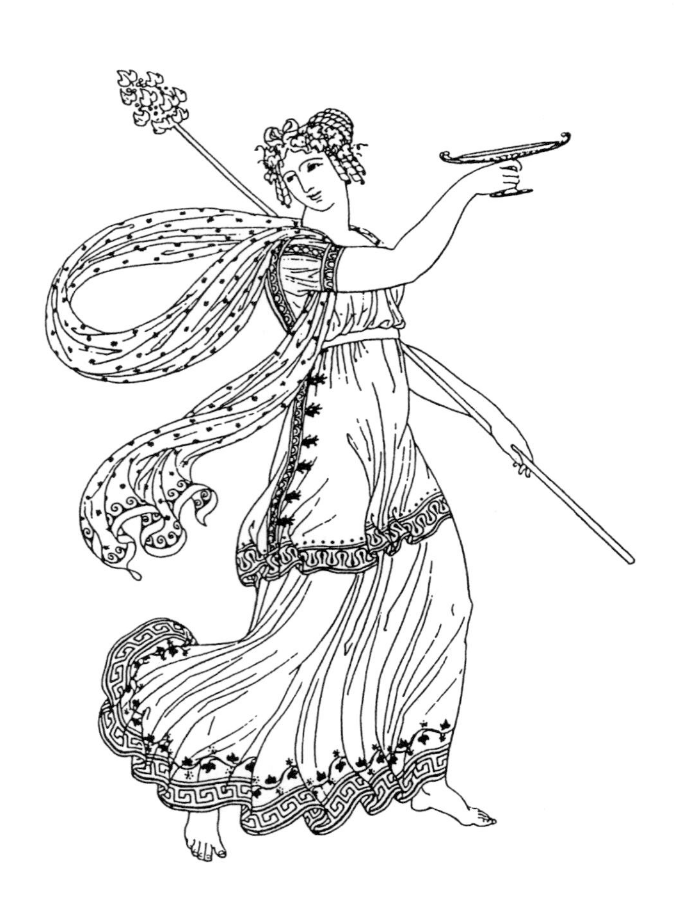

Castor Oil Packs

Castor oil packs assist enemas in cleansing and clearing the bowels. The absorption of the Castor oil through skin pores into the lymph system softens, relaxes and nourishes the bowels, as well as balancing the sympathetic and parasympathetic nervous systems, when it is absorbed into the lacteals in the small intestine. It also disperses congestion, relieves tension and helps to release any blockages or bowel pockets.

Dr. Raymond Christopher states in his book *School of Natural Healing*: "Castor oil helps to get rid of hardened mucus in the body, which may appear as cysts, tumors or polyps." Many patients resist this treatment because they fear it will be messy. When they finally do it and are rewarded by the results, they always wish they had done it earlier. Follow these instructions:

1. To prevent stains, place a towel over a piece of plastic to protect the chair or the bed.
2. Cover a cookie tin, or similar flat surface, with a plastic baggie.
3. Place a white cotton cloth or dish towel (no dyed colors) over the baggie.
4. Pour warmed Castor oil over the cloth, soaking it thoroughly without making it too wet. Fold the cloth to spread the oil evenly and then unfold it fully onto the plastic which has been placed on the cookie tin.
5. Cover the oil–soaked cloth with a second water moistened cotton cloth.
6. Cover these two layers of cloth with another baggie or piece of plastic. Lift them all off the bottom plastic bag, turn and place the Castor oil cloth directly on the skin. The moist cotton cloth remains in the middle with a baggie on top, so the final layer of thick towel will not be stained by the oil. Sometimes the oil runs out the side as the heat increases, so make sure the surface you are sitting or lying on is well protected as suggested above. The layers from the skin out are: oil–soaked cloth, damp cloth, plastic baggie and then the towel.
7. Place the heating pad over all of this. Hot water bottles can also be used but they are not so convenient because they are heavy, cool quickly and need refilling during the treatment. Don't fill hot water bottles too full, or they will feel heavy and uncomfortable, and will not lie flat on the abdomen.
8. Cover everything with another thick towel or blanket which wraps around the body to hold everything in place and to help retain the heat.
9. Enjoy this soothing and relaxing pack for one–and–one–half hours, three days in a row. Each day place the two layers of cotton and the top layer of plastic back on the protective layer of plastic on the cookie tin, then roll it up and put it away. Put new Castor oil on the cloth each time you apply it, taking care not to make it too oily.
10. For the next three days, massage the entire abdominal area with olive oil.
11. Wash the cloths and leave them in the sun and air to purify for at least one day.
12. Rest on the seventh day. Repeat the entire procedure again.

Enjoy the Castor oil pack by reading, writing, resting, meditating, watching television or videos, or sleeping while the pack is on. The relaxation of the solar plexus is very soothing, and especially valuable to release the kind of constipation caused by muscular tension. Make a strong effort to overcome any resistance to doing the Castor oil pack, and include it in any home care program.

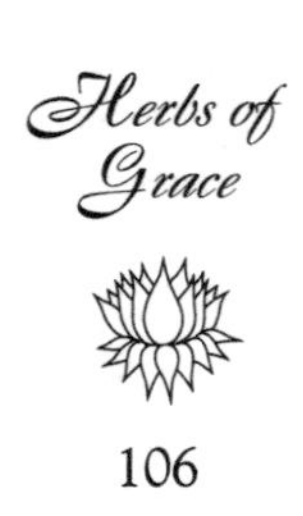

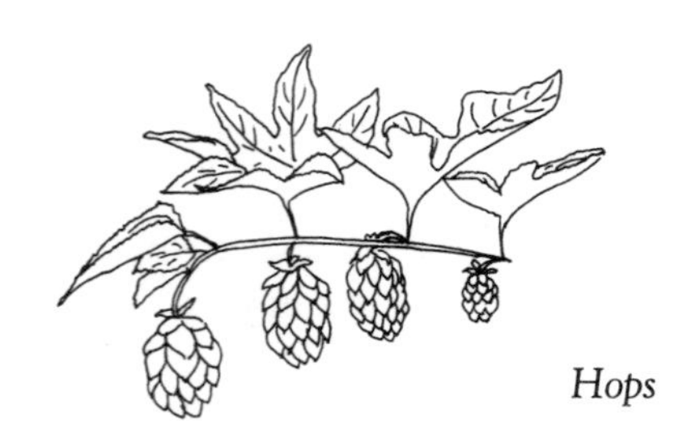

Hops

ENEMAS

There is so much emphasis in current fashion on external appearance that the mere mention of the word "enema" invokes expressions of repulsion or embarrassment. The yogis of old who maintained equilibrium between inner and outer cleanliness, in a detached manner, always included enema techniques in their lifestyle. Ancient yogic and ayurvedic texts, and the Essene Gospel of Peace include detailed information on methods of internal bowel cleansing.

In modern times the science of iridology helps to prove the relationship of the colon to disease, toxins and symptoms. Essentially, the colon is a hub. Each segment of the bowel has intricate multitudinous connections of circulation, lymph and nerves, which connect to specific reflex areas throughout the entire body. If one area of the colon is toxic, spastic or inflamed, the symptoms are not only found in the bowel itself, but also in the reflex area.

During surgery poisonous toxic conditions that exist inside the bowel and pollute the body via the bloodstream can be viewed first hand, yet their cause and effect, in terms of creating or increasing diseased conditions, are not considered or treated. The colon is supposed to serve as a reservoir from which the blood absorbs nutrients to circulate throughout the entire system. But when the colon is toxic, or impacted with fecal matter, poisons are distributed instead. Also, the afflicted person is not satisfied by normal food, feels hungry and eats much more than he needs because the nutrients are not absorbed and circulated, causing further stress on the body.

When people are asked if they are constipated they often immediately say no. On further discussion it is found that this denial can mean anything from one bowel movement daily, to every three days, or even once a week! Their doctors even consider this normal. Does it follow that if food is taken three times or more a day that it should be eliminated only once a day, or even less? Children with relaxed healthy systems usually have about three movements per day. If food is allowed to remain inside the bowel for longer than twelve hours it begins to deteriorate. Imagine how much more putrefactive it becomes if it remains in the bowel for twenty–four hours, or three days! Gas is manufactured and pressure causes further problems as the colon develops swellings and pockets which hold further deposits of toxic waste. Poisons from these toxic areas are carried throughout the entire system, causing toxemia.

Almost every person needs bowel cleansing. Once the bowel function is restored a regular maintenance program is advised. Just as a house requires spring cleaning and a car regular tune–ups, the bowel needs maintenance cleansing so that toxic wastes do not increase.

Effective bowel cleansing, rejuvenation and maintenance requires a combination of herbs, diet and massage, as well as packs and poultices. Enemas are also a significant supplemental aid that serves an important function in any bowel program. The various kinds of enemas and their suggested use are given on the next few pages.

How To Do an Enema

An enema should be a simple and pleasant experience. Collect the equipment and ingredients, prepare the enema fluid, set aside a relaxed half hour, pour an aromatherapy bath of Chamomile, Rosemary, Sandalwood and Lavender, provide reading material, music, candles and incense to create a nourishing and relaxing atmosphere. A gravity flow enema bucket or bag and two pints of enema fluid is required

Many people prefer to take their enema while they are soaking in a warm bath. Others prefer to lie on a towel, so that they can rise up into the yoga shoulder stand or the plow posture while the enema is retained. Others choose the use of a slant–board, allowing gravity to aid retention. It helps to have a hook in a convenient place from which to hang the enema bag or bucket. A simple hook can easily be made from a clothes hanger which can be hung over the shower head or water taps.

Once the organization is complete lubricate the enema tip with soap, vaseline, or oil, lie down on the right side and press the tip of the enema tube into the rectum until it is firmly in place. Release the tube lock, and let the liquid begin to flow inside. It is best to have the liquid at room temperature, as hot water will be uncomfortable, and cold water is harder to retain. Control the flow by stopping and starting as needed, and massaging the abdomen to help the fluid move by blockages. When all the fluid is inserted, lie quietly or rise up into the shoulder stand. Ideally, a person should be able to inject and retain a quart of fluid for at least ten minutes. Sometimes the urge to release cannot be ignored, and it is wise to let it go and begin all over again. As the bowel relaxes and clears, it is easier to receive and retain the liquid with a minimum of discomfort.

The enema liquid flows up the descending colon across the transverse, and down the ascending colon, so it is helpful to change positions during the enema procedure and massage the abdominal area. When a strong urge to release comes, it usually lasts only for a minute. Try to breathe quickly while turning both feet quickly in circles until the urge passes. Remember, the more the positive assistance of the enema is needed, the more the bowels will try to reject the enema fluid prematurely.

Each time an enema is administered, try to hold it longer than the time before. Remain lying on the right side or in the inverted posture. Once the benefits of enemas is experienced, do not be tempted to overuse them. Overuse of enemas can cause weakening of bowel tone and action, so it is important to realize when enemas should and should not be used. The cause of constipation must be relieved by applying discipline to overcome poor diet and exercise habits.

The most important benefit of enemas is the contribution they bring to body purification. Whenever any fasting or dietary changes release extra toxins into the liver, bowels, blood and lymph, enemas help remove them from the body. It is also a necessary part of any program dedicated to bowel cleansing. However, once the cleansing goal is achieved, the enema should be used only on a maintenance basis, sometimes once a week, once a month. They may also be used whenever there are colds, flu, infections or digestive problems. If constipation persists, use internal herbal formulae, apply Castor oil packs, make dietary changes and seek professional guidance. Do not avoid curing the cause of constipation or diarrhea by abusing the use of enemas.

Different Types of Enemas

Plain Water Enema

A warm water enema will effectively cleanse the bowels and release toxins that may be causing headaches and flatulence. Its effects are superficial but can be relied on whenever any of the other enema teas of liquids are not readily available.

Herbal Enemas

Make a strong infusion of herbal teas or a decoction of roots and barks. Strain and cool. Use two teaspoons of herbs per pint of water, four teaspoons for each quart. Make the enema in advance, but use within twenty–four hours. The decoction should be kept in a glass container in a refrigerator or a cool place. Make herbal infusions or decoctions in stainless steel or glass pots.

Catnip Enema	Mildly nervine, calming, soothing, relaxing; effectively brings down fevers; excellent for use with hysterical or upset children
Chamomile Enema	Excellent for recuperative periods after illness or a healing crisis; calming and soothing
Detoxifying Enema	Make a decoction of Yellow Dock and Burdock roots, then add a Red Clover and Red Raspberry infusion; this enema stimulates the liver to dump bile, relieving stress and pain in a healing crisis
Slippery Elm Enema	A mucilaginous, soothing, softening and nourishing enema; good for irritation, discomfort or whenever there is difficulty eating or retaining food; the bowel directly absorbs the nutrients
Sage Enema	Warming, purifying
Garlic Injection	Profoundly purifying, this is an excellent aid in the treatment of worms; liquidize four cloves Garlic in one pint of warm water, strain; do not use if there are hemorrhoids or sensitive skin; inject into the rectum with a bowel syringe
Astringent Enema	Witch Hazel, Bayberry or White Oak bark are used to help stop diarrhea and dysentery
Flaxseed Enema	Relieves inflammation, pain and bleeding; add two teaspoons liquid chlorophyll to speed in the healing process
Wheatgrass Implant	Inject one–quarter to one–half cup pure chlorophyll wheatgrass juice after the bowel has been cleansed with a plain water enema, to restore positivity to the bowel and blood stream; excellent for chronic disease; for even better results mix equally with Rejuvelac – which is water that has been soaked in wheat overnight

Coffee Enemas

The coffee enema is widely publicized these days as an important part of cancer therapy and chronic care naturopathy. It is excellent to relieve healing crisis pain and discomfort, to stimulate the liver to release bile, and to encourage deep cleansing of the colon by stimulating peristaltic activity. It is a regular part of both the Gerson cancer therapy and the Kelly cancer program.

Using organic coffee only, the enema is prepared by putting three tablespoons of ground, unprocessed, preferably organic coffee into one quart of distilled water which has just been brought to a boil. Continue boiling for three minutes, then simmer on very low heat for twenty minutes. Wash the bowel first with one or two plain water enemas. Cool, strain and inject the fluid when it reaches body temperature. Retain ten to fifteen minutes. This can be used every morning when on a detoxification program or fast, and every hour during an acute healing crisis. The bowels continue to operate independently even when taking the coffee enema regularly, and begin functioning on their own after it is discontinued. The coffee enema is recommended following a lymph massage to cleanse the colon after the lymph has drained into the bowel. The coffee enema is not recommended before sleep as it is too stimulating.

An herbal substitute for the coffee enema is a decoction of Red Clover blossoms, Yellow Dock root, Burdock and Red Raspberry leaves. This works as effectively as the coffee enema with the added benefit of herbal nutrients. It is also less stimulating and is especially recommended when the coffee enema has to be done at night. I created this formula when I adjusted the Gerson cancer program for use with vegetarian clients. This formula received the approval of Margaret Strauss, granddaughter of Max Gerson, after I discussed it with her in England.

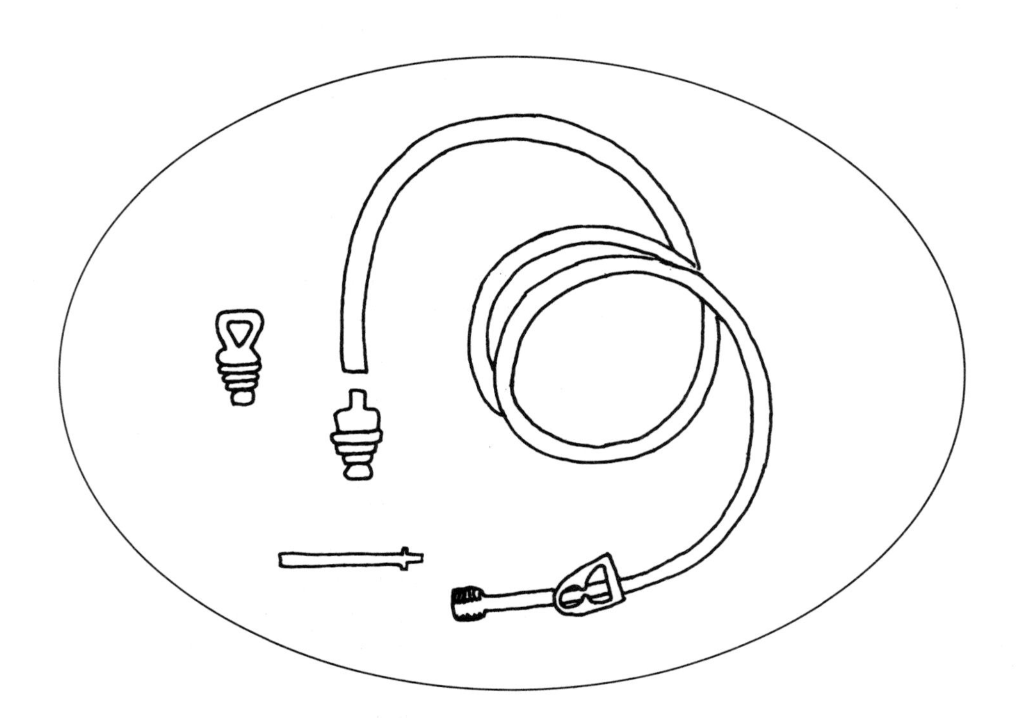

Spirulina Enemas

The use of Spirulina plankton enemas, together with fasting and purification programs, is an excellent way to cleanse the colon and purify the blood stream as quickly as possible. Spirulina has the unique advantage of supplying strength and power through the absorption of the plankton into the bowel wall at the same time as softening impacted fecal matter and stimulating peristalsis. The direct nutrition absorbed by the colon provides proteins and essential amino acids, laying a balanced foundation for purification, as hunger and weakness are prevented by the Spirulina. Clear the colon first by using one or more plain water enemas. When the bowel is quite empty inject the spirulina enema and retain as long as possible. Instructions for the Spirulina enema are as follows:

1. Heat one blender full of distilled water to body temperature.

2. Mix two teaspoons Spirulina powder with a small amount of cold water until it forms a smooth paste.

3. Add two teaspoons vegetable glycerin and stir together.

4. Add this loose paste to a blender half full of the warm distilled water and mix at slow speed.

5. Add the remaining distilled water slowly, filling the blender.

6. Fill the enema bag with the mixture and use immediately.

This method will cleanse the lower and upper bowel with spirulina and encourage a complete peristaltic downward action. The plankton is also absorbed into the bowel wall, helping to soften, loosen and eliminate toxic bowel residue.

Inject the mixture a little at a time while lying on the right side. Roll back and forth from the left to the right side, and massage the bowel area. If you feel that retention is impossible, then eject, and start the process over again. With practice the bowel becomes accustomed to the enemas, and eventually you will be able to retain a full enema of two quarts for five to ten minutes while massaging the abdomen. The yoga shoulder stand will help the spirulina to reach the full length of the large intestine, including the bottom of the ascending colon.

Vegetable glycerin helps to emulsify the mixture, soften the impacted faeces and lubricate the walls of the colon. Take the enema the first night of any fast, and for the next two nights. While you continue the fast, take one every other day. After the fast take a Spirulina enema once a month on a regular basis for effective bowel maintenance. Use Spirulina powder that does not have any additives or fillers.

Enema Equipment

Enema or Douche Bucket

Enema buckets are non–brittle, white plastic, and have a 1.2 liter or two pint capacity. They come complete with tube and nozzles. The bucket has a hook hole on one side to hang it on a wall–mounted hook. Oils and herbs can easily be cleaned out of the bucket.

Enema or Douche Bag

The bag is collapsible and has a two quart capacity. It has a reinforced top for mounting on a small hook. Easily cleaned inside, it packs into a small bag for both home and travel use. It comes complete with enema and douche nozzles.

Enema or Douche Hot Water Bottle

The water bottle combination provides the necessary tube, clip, enema and douche nozzles to be used with a hot water bottle. It is useful for home and travel, especially if you want to use a hot water bottle for a Castor oil pack or to keep warm during cold weather. The disadvantage is that you can't clean it as thoroughly or as easily of herbs and powders. It is fine for enemas made from warm water or well–strained herbal teas.

Rectal Syringe

The rectal syringe is a squeezable rubber bulb with a nozzle. It is useful for rectal implants, but generally it doesn't hold enough fluid for an efficient enema, and doesn't get the fluid far enough into the large intestine. Gravity flow enema kits are best.

Rectal Implant Tube

A useful addition to any of the above, is a soft, flexible 14–inch rectal implant tube with two laterally positioned end holes, rather than a single one in the end that may get blocked. This releases the enema fluid higher into the colon so that the fluid goes more completely into the ascending colon. It fits all the enema kits, slipping over the standard rectal nozzle, and makes the insertion of the enema nozzle smoother and easier.

One of the pleasant results of a clean colon is a more stable emotional life. It is recognized among natural healers that a constipated person is an irritable, impatient one. If we could only realize consciously the importance of the effect of internal hygiene on general health, well–being and appearance, we would balance all our efforts for external appearance with internal cleanliness. It is certainly an essential aspect of any body cleansing program, whether for preventive or curative treatment. Give it a place along with other beauty and health routines. Become familiar with enemas so that they can be applied comfortably whenever they are needed. Many people have a resistance toward enemas, and we hope this information will help you to overcome this. Your life will benefit from applying these self–treatments when appropriate.

FLOWER REMEDIES

Bach Flower Remedies

The thirty–eight remedies used in this method of treatment are all prepared from the flowers of wild plants, bushes and trees and none of them are harmful or habit–forming. They are potentized, etheric, vibrational, natural medicines to restore equilibrium within the life of the patient. They are prescribed, not directly for the physical complaint, but for the sufferer's mental and emotional state – worry, fear, depression, irritability, etc. – because these indulgent or negative states of mind and moods not only hinder recovery of health and retard convalescence but are the primary causes of sickness and disease.

Any long or continued worry or fear will deplete the individual's vitality and cause the person to feel out of sorts, below par or not themselves. The body then loses its natural resistance to disease and becomes prey to infection and illness, whether it be the common cold, digestive disturbances or more chronic diseases. It is the sufferer of the illness who needs treatment, not the complaint. As peace and harmony return to the mind, health will also return to the body.

This method of treatment and the remedies were discovered by a medical doctor who had practiced for over twenty years in London as a Harley Street consultant, bacteriologist and homeopath. The late Edward Bach, M.B., B.S., M.R.C.S., L.R.C.P., D.P.H., gave up his lucrative practice in 1930 to devote himself to full–time research work to seek remedies in the plant world that would restore vitality to the sick, so that the sufferers themselves would be able to overcome their worry, fear and depression and assist in their own healing.

Inspiring quotations from Dr. Bach's book *Heal Thyself* are:

"What we know as disease is an ultimate result produced in the body, the end product of deep and long acting forces..."

"Disease is in essence the result of conflict between Soul and Mind and will never be eradicated except by spiritual and mental effort."

"... disease, though apparently so cruel, is in itself beneficent and for our good and, if rightly interpreted, it will guide us to our essential faults. If properly treated it will be the cause of the removal of those faults and leave us better and greater then before. Suffering is a corrective to point out a lesson which by other means we have failed to grasp, and never can it be eradicated until that lesson is learned."

The practitioner prescribes a personalized remedy after a visit with the patient. The patient accepts the diagnosis of the practitioner, but is not told which particular remedies have been prescribed because any mental thoughts directed to those remedies will disturb the healing process.

California Flower Remedies

California flower remedies continue the tradition of the Bach flower remedies. They are in tune with the spirit of this age and resonate with increased mental and spiritual sensitivity. Their essences open and clear areas such as creativity, emotions, negativity, sexuality (balancing male and female principles) and spirituality, and provide the strength to overcome obstacles.

Other Flower Essences

Every year more flower essences are being created. Sets are now available of local plants from Alaska, Australia and Hawaii, as well as from other areas of the world, or from specialized gardens. The testimonies of their effectiveness are sincere and enthusiastic. Try different systems, or try them all! Purchase sets from health food stores, herbal suppliers or from ads in herbal or health magazines. These sets enable individuals to mix their own formulae as well as to share them with family and friends. Dr. Bach's dream was for people to be able to help themselves. There is also a Rocky Mountain flower essence company in Boulder, Colorado which provides a seven chakra flower essence kit as well as essences for personal spiritual evolution.

Bach Flower Remedy Dosage

1. *Emergency Conditions:* Take four drops in water every sixty seconds. Massage the head, hands and feet, or the entire body with water which has at least twelve drops of the remedy dissolved in it. Immerse in a flower remedy bath to relieve convulsions, accident, shock or lightning strikes. Gradually increase the time between doses as the condition improves. Seek professional help as quickly as possible.

2. *Acute Conditions:* As the person recovers, lengthen the time between doses to every half hour, then switch to hourly doses until the condition improves.

3. *Purification, Regeneration, Transformation Programs:* Take hourly for five to seven days during waking hours, then four times daily as required.

4. *Long term treatment to achieve mental and emotional balance and neutralize personality excesses or shortages*: Take four to six times daily, especially on waking and before sleep.

Important Hints for Taking the Bach Flower Remedies

1. Do not touch the tongue with the dropper. If this happens, disinfect the dropper with boiling water before putting back into the bottle. Do not contaminate the dropper with saliva.

2. Always take the remedy upon waking and just before sleep.

3. Divide the remedy into two bottles. Keep one at home and keep one in a purse or pocket, so that it is readily available at work or on the go.

Making Your Own Remedies From Stock Bottles

If you wish you can purchase your own stock bottles of individual remedies or a full set from a health food store or a herbal catalogue so that you can make your own remedies. Make sure you also purchase books or literature to study the remedies first. Once you have decided what you wish to take, mix the remedies into your dropper bottle in the following way:

1. Buy a one–ounce dropper bottle from the drug store or chemist and sterilize.

2. Fill it nearly full with pure well water or bottled spring water. Do not use mineral or distilled water unless it has been poured through the air to energize it. Store it in sunlight in a glass bottle for further energizing. Do not use tap water because its chemicals will alter the sensitive homeopathic flower remedy.

3. Drop four drops from each individual remedy into the water in the one–ounce bottle. This mixture is the individual prescription. Follow the dosage instructions above.

4. The master stock bottles of the individual remedies may be stored indefinitely as they are preserved in a brandy base. However, don't keep bottles in direct sunlight or in heat.

5. There is no need to add brandy to your prescription bottle unless you are in a very hot climate. If the remedy ever tastes odd, pour it out, sterilize the bottle, and start over with a fresh remedy.

6. We recommend that you always keep *Rescue Remedy* on hand for emergencies in a home medicine chest, in the car and in your travel bag.

7. Remember that the remedies are absorbed into the central nervous system through the palette. It is essential to hold the remedy in the mouth for at least thirty to sixty seconds. Mix it with saliva, swish it around a few times and then swallow. If it is swallowed immediately, there will be little benefit from the remedies.

8. The mouth should be clean. Don't take the remedies with food, or immediately before or after drinking any other liquids or brushing the teeth.

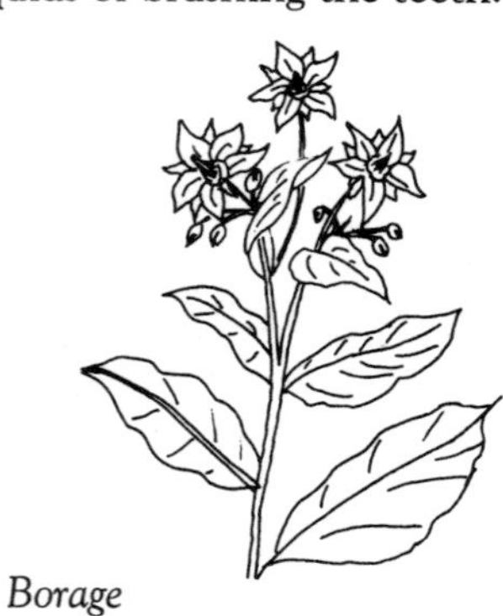

Borage

Fomentations

Fomentations are particularly useful for overnight treatments, or if a condition requires treatment over a large body area.

Using proportions of one teaspoon of powdered herb per cup of water, make up enough strong herbal infusion or decoction to soak enough 100% cotton cloths (old sheets or dishcloths are good) to cover the required body area. Pour boiling water over the herbs which are contained in a cloth bag. Place the cloths in the herbal mixture. Infuse, stirring occasionally until at least one hour has passed. If the mixture is cool, add a little boiling water. Wring out and remove the cloths. Wrap them around the body part, and secure with a stretch bandage. Make sure the bed is protected with towels and a plastic sheet so the herbs do not stain the sheets.

Varicose Vein Fomentations

When treating varicose veins with an infusion of witch hazel, soak fine cotton, linen, or silk in the infusion, and wrap the cloth around the legs. Put stockings over the wraps, and wear pants or a long skirt. The effect of this nutrient over the days and nights will make a strong contribution to the effectiveness of any internal herbal and dietary treatment. Body heat dries out the cloths, and they have to be moistened regularly and replaced every twelve hours. Use different cloths for each application. Wash and hang the used cloths in the sun and air both to freshen them and to release negative energy.

Skin Disease Fomentations

Whenever chronic eczema and psoriasis, or acute conditions such as poison oak or poison ivy create severe itching, use fomentations to relieve and heal these conditions. Make a large pot of several handfuls of infused Chickweed herb, strain and pour in a bath. Put cotton cloths in the bath, soak them thoroughly and then apply as needed, remoistening them several times during the day, and before sleep. Prepare fresh herbs every twenty–four hours.

The bath can also be used for a therapeutic herbal soak any time during the night or day. At the same time take herbs internally to release the cause of the condition. Whatever is good for you internally will be good externally, so any of the internal herbs or formulae can also be prepared as an infusion to be used for baths and fomentations. Hand and foot baths quickly absorb the healing chemistry of herbs directly into the capillary circulation and lymphatic fluids, increasing the speed of recovery. This is particularly useful whenever weakness or debilitation makes the digestion of herbs and food difficult.

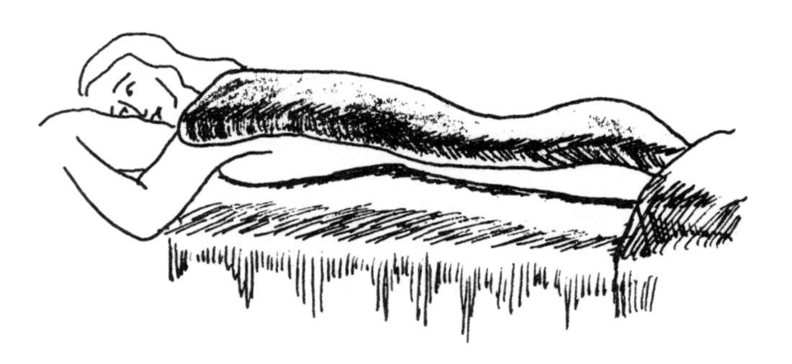

Gall Bladder Cleanse

The treatment outlined below has been developed from several sources. The first inspiration was from Frank Robert's excellent book *Modern Herbalism for Digestive Disorders*. Once his ideas were integrated into my holistic natural healing practice and guided by iridology, the cleanse was placed within a framework of preparation, administration and follow up. This treatment was tested for several months by hundreds of people at the Alive Polarity communities in Washington and California. There both staff and students participated in gall bladder cleanses during the purifying week of their basic program. Time and again, this safe method gives excellent results as the release of crystallization on the physical level open the way for transformation on the emotional and mental levels.

Gall Bladder Cleanse Needs

* 1/4 to 1/2 cup cold–pressed, high quality, pure olive oil
* 1/2 to 1 cup fresh squeezed lemon juice
* enema kit
* strainer screen, flour sifter or large tea strainer
* coffee enema or herbal detoxifying enema ingredients (see Enema section)

Gall Bladder Cleanse Instructions

1. Choose a weekend, or two days, when you do not have any social engagements or commitments, especially on the second day.

2. Eat a light, fresh fruit or vegetable salad for lunch, and drink juices and herb teas. Do not eat anything after the midday meal on the first day. The cleanse is best when prepared for and administered after a juice fast or purifying diet.

3. Commence treatment about 7 p.m.

4. Take four tablespoons of olive oil, immediately followed by one or more tablespoons of fresh undiluted, unsweetened lemon juice. This will reduce the effect of the oil and clear the mouth. Take the oil in one quick swallow. Hold your breath and your nose to reduce the sense of smell and follow quickly with the lemon juice. Keep your mind uplifted and on other things. Music, television or videos are entertaining diversions.

5. Repeat every fifteen minutes until all the oil is taken. Take extra tablespoons of lemon juice as needed to help settle the stomach and to remove excess oil from the mouth.

6. Between each dose, lie on the right side with the head on a pillow, with the knees bent toward the chest. At the Alive Polarity community the cleanse was administered to groups of fifteen to twenty people at the same time. Curled together, all lying on our right side on cushions on the floor, we looked like a group of sardines as we watched a video. Group support is wonderful, especially if it is the first time that you are doing this cleanse.

7. Add the beauty of the ether element to this treatment. Use a clear glass punch bowl to display the golden liquid olive oil, and a crystal pitcher for the lemon juice. Drink out of wine glasses and celebrate the positivity that is being given.

8. The treatment can also be successful with only one–half pint of olive oil, especially when there is not a chronic gall stone condition.

9. For chronic gall stone conditions, prepare for the treatment by following the purifying diet for at least one week, doing reflexology foot massage especially on the liver/gall bladder area, applying the Castor oil pack over the liver/gall bladder area for three days before the cleanse. Practice relaxation, use poultices, and take herbal baths, enemas, massage and Bach flower remedies before the gall bladder cleanse. A tight, tense, congested gall bladder area will make the treatment more uncomfortable than it needs to be. If a clear elimination is to take place, all these other dimensions of holistic healing need to be applied first.

10. Lie down for one hour after the last dose has been taken.

11. Retire early. Drink herb teas or water, but do not eat for the remainder of the first day or on the second day.

Possible Reactions to the Gall Bladder Cleanse

Nausea: if any oil is vomited, continue taking the doses. Overcome any resistance. Nausea begins in the mind. Breathe deeply. Suck on a lemon. Take the mind off your stomach. Staying quiet and still will reduce nausea. If you vomit some of the oil, don't worry about it. Relax and watch a video, or read quietly.

Gas: to reduce gas, rub your stomach and rock in a squatting position, gently, moving back and forth. Drink Wild Yam root tea.

Burning: burning during bowel movements means that chemical toxins are being released from the liver. Do not worry. Gerson Therapy clients have observed this reaction also, and they confirm that the release of chemicals is often accompanied by slight burning sensations.

Sleeplessness: often people experience a happy, high feeling. Some dream a lot. Others sleep soundly. If you do this treatment more than once, you will find that each time the experience is different, depending on what the body is releasing with the cleanse.

Whenever there is an urge to move the bowels, pass the movement into a wire mesh strainer. Rinse water over the bowel matter, so that only stones and gravel remain. Collect the stones and gravel, so you can see what has been released. I have even seen small tumors released. The stones vary in color and size. The usual color is the green biliverdin bile pigment. On occasion red bilirubin stones are passed. Usually white calcareous gall stones will not pass with

this cleanse. They need to be dissolved from within by the Hydrangea root kidney stone cleanse described in the Herbal and Naturopathy Treatments chapter. Take the coffee or herbal detoxifying enema the following morning to stimulate elimination.

The stones come out up to forty–eight hours after the cleanse, and as soon as they are exposed to the atmosphere they begin to soften, and eventually completely dissolve. In some cases the liquifying takes place before they leave the bowel. In this case the bowel movement is very soft and oily. Often one–half to one cup of stones of varying bean, seed or gravel sizes are passed. They dissolve over a couple of days. If you want to show them to your doctor, take them to his office right away or photograph them immediately, placed next to a ruler to show their size.

Follow up to the Gall Bladder Cleanse

1. Repeat the cleanse in three months.

2. Minimize or eliminate fats, fried foods and dairy products in the diet.

3. It is important to follow the cleanse with a course of the Gall Bladder formula, to clear the tissue sensitivity and reduce inflammation. This formula should be taken for a minimum of six weeks and preferably for about twelve weeks after the cleanse.

4. Explore emotional causes for gall stones. Use the Bach flower remedies or other flower essences, together with counselling, to clear negative emotions such as anger, fear, resentment, jealousy and bitterness.

Individual Responses to the Gall Bladder Cleanse

Most people experience a release. Some describe a feeling of lightness and joy. Freeing the gall bladder from crystallization will lighten the emotions as well as the physical body.

Healing Crisis or Achievement ?

Healing Achievement

This system of natural medicine eliminates the need for dramatic and uncomfortable healing crises because our balanced individualized treatment activates all the eliminative channels and releases toxins on a daily basis rather than collecting them for release all at once. As long as a reaction does not last longer than three days, consider it a healing achievement. Consult and communicate with your practitioner and receive guidance as to how to support this energetic healing process.

Symptoms and Discomforts

When you have any discomfort such as rashes, fevers, diarrhea, nausea or rough spots during any treatment, re–read this section. Go to bed if necessary. Take a coffee or detoxifying enema. Have a stimulating bath of Mustard, Cayenne and Ginger powder, a sauna or a Turkish bath. Scrub your skin thoroughly. Have a massage. Stimulate reflexology pressure points. Have an aromatherapy, herbal or Epsom salts bath. Go through rough periods using natural methods, and conserve energy for the healing process.

Do Not Suppress

Do not take aspirin, antibiotics or suppressive medications of any kind. While healing crises may be uncomfortable they should not be unduly difficult. There is much that can be done to minimize any discomfort.

Cleansing Cycles

Cleansing often takes place in cycles of seven days, seven weeks, seven months, or even seven years. It is important to understand that what appears to be an illness can actually be caused by the strengthening of the body. Old illnesses or symptoms reappear, stay around for one to three days, then disappear. This is an excellent sign, showing evidence that the healing reversal process is taking place. Congratulations. If the eliminative organs have been prepared to handle the healing crisis, most boils, rashes, pain, headaches or diarrhea can be avoided or experienced only minimally.

Quotes from Practitioners

"*A healing crisis is an acute reaction resulting from the ascendancy of Nature's healing forces over disease conditions. Its tendency is toward recovery and it is therefore in conformity with Nature's constructive principle.*" – Dr. Henry Lindlahr

"*There are three stages through which a person must pass in getting well. They are the eliminative, the transitional and the building stages. The crisis usually occurs during the transitional period, which is the time when the new tissue has matured sufficiently to take on the functions of a more perfect body.*"
– Dr. Bernard Jensen

"*All cure starts from within out and from the head down and in reverse order as the symptoms have appeared.*" – Hering's Law of Cure

Support Your Body To Do Its Work

Let the body do its work unhampered. It is at this time that the patient and the practitioner stand by and support nature as it takes its course. Encourage elimination. Relax instead of react. This is what you have been working for. Make the most of it, because it will pass away very soon. Work with it. Learn how to ease your body through these active eliminations by using natural methods.

HERPES

The treatment and cure of herpes can be a delicate, long–term process. Because the virus feeds on toxic matter and rises to ascendancy during periods of stress or exhaustion, cure involves strong purification together with nourishing, strengthening herbs based on iridology readings, which reveal the condition of eliminative channels and major organs and body systems. When strong efforts are made to administer the treatment over a period of six months, symptoms disappear, or reappear in a very slight form only when undue stress or fatigue is unavoidable.

It is essential to adjust living habits. Strict efforts must be kept up for several months. When the system is cleansed, patients can resume some of their previous habits. However, the condition is often the result of living habits, so the cause and effect pattern needs to be recognized and changed.

Avoid: sugar, animal protein, fish, eggs, white flour products, coffee, tea, cigarettes, alcohol, drugs and dairy products.

Clothing: wear only 100% cotton or silk underwear and loose trousers or skirts to allow air to circulate and to minimize irritation.

Daily Habits

1. Wash the genitals before and after passing water or bowel movements
2. Sunbathe the genitals whenever possible
3. Get adequate rest, and enough sleep; keep regular hours
4. Do not have sex when you have a sore or irritation
5. Disinfect hands after touching sores or genitals
6. Boil or disinfect underwear and wash separately

Herbal Program for Herpes

Although individual assessment with iridology is recommended, a general program for at least six months consists of the following formulae for systemic treatment:

1. Bowel Rejuvenator formula
2. Antibiotics Naturally formula
3. Nerve Rejuvenator formula
4. Blood Purifying formula

Herbal Treatment for Acute Herpes

1. Echinacea – 2 capsules every 2 hours
2. Four to six cups of Sarsaparilla tea daily
3. Chronic Purifier formula – one capsule every two hours
4. Two to three ounces of wheatgrass juice daily
5. The juicy wheatgrass pulp can also be applied directly on the genitals

Vitamins for Herpes

1. 2000 mg. vitamin C daily
2. Vitamin B complex
3. Vitamin A
4. Eight to twelve capsules of Kelp daily
5. Take regular doses of bee pollen which is high in amino acids

Treatment For Herpes Sores

1. Aloe Vera gel
2. Chickweed ointment for itching
3. Comfrey ointment for healing
4. Balm of Gilead for healing
5. Vitamin E oil or wheat germ oil for soothing and healing
6. Three to four drops of Myrrh tincture, three to four times a day, or after passing water; this is antiseptic and gives immediate relief

Amino Acids for Herpes

1. *Tryptophan*
   Take one tablet before retiring when you feel the herpes coming on
2. *Lysine*
   Take 1500 mg. daily – lesions usually disappear overnight
   Take 500 mg. daily as a maintenance dose

Sitz Baths for Herpes

Simmer one–quarter cup of Uva Ursi for thirty minutes in two quarts of water. Dilute into a lukewarm bath and sit in it for thirty minutes, keeping the upper part of your body and knees out of the water. Add more warm water if the bath gets too cool. Apply Myrrh tincture or any of the suggested ointments to the sores after showers or baths.

Life Style Changes for Herpes

Whenever irritating symptoms occur in any body area there are life lessons to be learned. Herpes sufferers have to face their emotional self and ask themselves what this disease is revealing about their lives. How are they creating it? What is its purpose? They have to look honestly at their sexual life. What changes do they need to make to bring about peace, contentment and balance, as well as physical healing? Stress also aggravates herpes.

True cure will only come when we are willing to face the truth of our own lives. We need to muster the essential discrimination to choose and follow through with a healthy lifestyle that will serve our highest purpose.

Kidney/Gall Stone Cleanse

Materials:

1. Two ounces Hydrangea root
2. One quart freshly extracted apple juice, or a pure commercial brand in a glass container.

Instructions:

1. Choose a cool room and let the Hydrangea root soak in the apple juice for three days. Shake the bottle three times a day. Begin a purifying diet.

2. Administer a Castor oil pack over the liver and gall bladder area and a Ginger poultice over the kidneys at night. Refer to the Herbal and Naturopathy Treatments chapter.

2. On the fourth day, simmer the mixture in a stainless steel pot, then set aside.

3. On the fifth day, start a juice cleanse. Refer to the Nourishment chapter.

4. Strain the Hydrangea mixture and take one ounce each waking hour until it is all consumed.

Follow up: drink only natural juices and distilled water to help avoid a recurrence of the stones. Take a minimum of eight glasses per day. Twelve glasses are preferred.

Repeat: two times a year for prevention and maintenance.

Reflexology: work on kidney reflexes for forty minutes, twenty on each foot using deep massage, gradually increasing the pressure as the condition clears.

Castor Oil Pack: use over the lower abdomen during the acute phase, then once a month for three months. This relieves painful congestion and helps to free the area so that it can release, heal and strengthen. Refer to the Herbal and Naturopathy Treatments chapter.

Herbal Teas: drink Waterbalance or Parsley herbal tea, at least three cups each day.

Bowels: deep cleansing with herbal formulae and softening with Castor oil packs will help to remove bowel pockets which may be spreading toxins to the kidney/bladder areas.

Diet: make a commitment to eat only a careful mucusless, vegetarian diet, with plenty of alkaline foods and fresh organic fruits and vegetables.

Caution: avoid mineral and tap water, inorganic minerals in supplements, aspirins and salt.

Kidney Ginger Poultice

This poultice is an excellent heating and stimulating treatment for the kidneys and adrenals. I have also used it in emergencies for injuries. Once in India when I pulled a muscle by running too fast, I used the fresh grated Ginger poultice and the injury was healed. I could walk without a limp by morning because all the pain was gone.

Finely grate fresh Ginger on two square gauze bandages. You will need enough of the soft, moist, freshly grated root to cover the kidney/adrenal area in the lower back. This area feels like a small hollow on either side of the spine. If you feel unsure about the location ask someone to help. Bend over and place the gauze bandages on the back with the Ginger next to the skin. Wrap with stretch bandages and secure. Use plastic and then a dark towel to lie on through the night to protect the bed. Do not wear any night clothes that will be ruined if moisture leaks out.

At times this pack will feel very hot. Do not worry. I have never known anyone who has been burned by a fresh Ginger poultice. It is best not to lie on the pack for any length of time as this increases the heat. The poultice will be dry in the morning. Remove it before bathing.

Poultices

Poultices provide direct nourishment to areas of need. Herbal nutrients are absorbed directly through the pores into the skin and then circulated to the needy glands, organs and tissues. This relieves the injured area from having to draw nutrient from other parts of the body through the blood and lymph contributing to congestion, inflammation, swelling and pain.

Internal herbal formulae can also be applied directly over the area as poultices. Respiratory herbs that are taken internally for bronchitis or asthma can also be applied as a poultice over the lungs. Broken bones, tissues, muscles and ligaments heal more quickly when the Body Building formula is placed over the injured area. Poultices offer outer support, direct feeding and the energetic effects of heating, cooling and drawing. The skin is used as a permeable membrane that absorbs the nutrients directly to areas of need. Although there are many types of poultices we have selected the most important groups, which are described below.

Many healers and herbalists do not utilize poultices, fomentations and herbal baths because they do not know their power, or they feel they are messy, time–consuming and require high quantities of herbs. Make the effort. Try the poultices. Experience their power. In my practice and through this book I always teach my clients and students the use of herbal and naturopathic home treatments to support their internal purification, regeneration and transformation.

In my early years of practice in England, I set aside three hours for every patient. While I took the case history and iris analysis they sat with their feet in a Lobelia foot bath to help them relax and to soften their feet. After the analysis I taught them the use of a poultice by doing the first one right then and there. While the poultice did its work I gave them a reflexology treatment. Continuous superb healing results built my practice and school. When enough time, love and care are combined with the full range of treatments, the results are beyond most people's expectations.

Different Types of Poultices

Cooling Poultices

Sunburn and mild burns can be effectively treated with frequent applications of Aloe Vera pulp applied directly on the skin. Best results are achieved with fresh Aloe Vera gel, but if this is not available, use pure commercial products available at health food stores. Cucumber is also an effective coolant. Do not use ice except in extreme emergencies. Wrap it well so that the extreme cold does not damage the skin.

Drawing Poultices

Whenever there are boils, insect or snake bites, blood poisoning, cysts or infections due to slivers, punctures, hang nails or swollen glands, herbal and vegetable poultices will help to draw the pus, foreign matter or poison so that it can be eliminated. The use of the wisdom herb, Lobelia, in the formula adds the intelligence necessary to guide the elimination to clear internally or externally, according to what is best for the body. Traditionally, onions, cabbage and other steamed or boiled vegetables produce an excellent drawing effect, as well as Mullein, Comfrey, Elecampagne and Marshmallow herbs.

Heating Poultices

Imbalances of circulation, emotional excess, stress and weather exposure are best treated with herbs that are warming, such as Ginger, Mustard and Cayenne. Grate fresh Ginger onto a gauze bandage for best results. Mustard requires care as it may burn the skin, so it needs to be wrapped and taken off from time to time to make sure aggravation does not occur. These herbs can also be mixed into baths for a general heat replenishment, to increase circulation, and to bring blood to the surface. Use short cold immersions or showers at the end of the treatment to restore the circulation to the core of the body, alkalinize the blood and increase energy.

Nourishing and Healing Poultices

Whenever there are injuries, sprains, wounds or broken bones, use herbal poultices to provide healing nutrients so that the body can repair quickly and easily without having to draw excess blood and lymph to the area, causing swelling, inflammation and pain. Comfrey, Elecampagne, Mullein, Marshmallow, Slippery Elm or wheatgrass are excellent for this purpose.

Softening Poultices

Poultices are also used to soften and relax areas that have become hardened, tense and toxic, such as breast lumps, glandular swellings and bowel pockets. Castor oil, Golden Seal, Slippery Elm, Lobelia, Mullein and Comfrey can be used individually or combined. The more you know the activities of individual herbs and the dynamics of a particular health condition, the more effectively you will be able to use individual or combined herbal poultice mixtures.

Swelling Poultices

Poultices made from Mullein, Lobelia, Slippery Elm, Comfrey and Golden Seal soften and disperse swollen glands, lumps or boils in the neck, groin, underarm, ears and other areas. They can be wrapped with stretch bandages to hold them in place. Apply a fresh poultice at night.

POULTICE FORMULAE

Breast lumps	3 parts Poke root and one part Slippery Elm
Burns and wounds	Comfrey root powder, honey and vitamin E oil
Fractures, sprains, injured muscles	Comfrey root, Body Building formula and Slippery Elm
Itching	3 parts Chickweed and one part Slippery Elm
Kidney, adrenal, lower back aches	Fresh grated Ginger root
Pain, congestion, respiratory distress, swellings	3 parts Lobelia, one part each of Slippery Elm and Mullein
Swollen glands	3 parts Mullein, and one part each of Lobelia and Slippery Elm

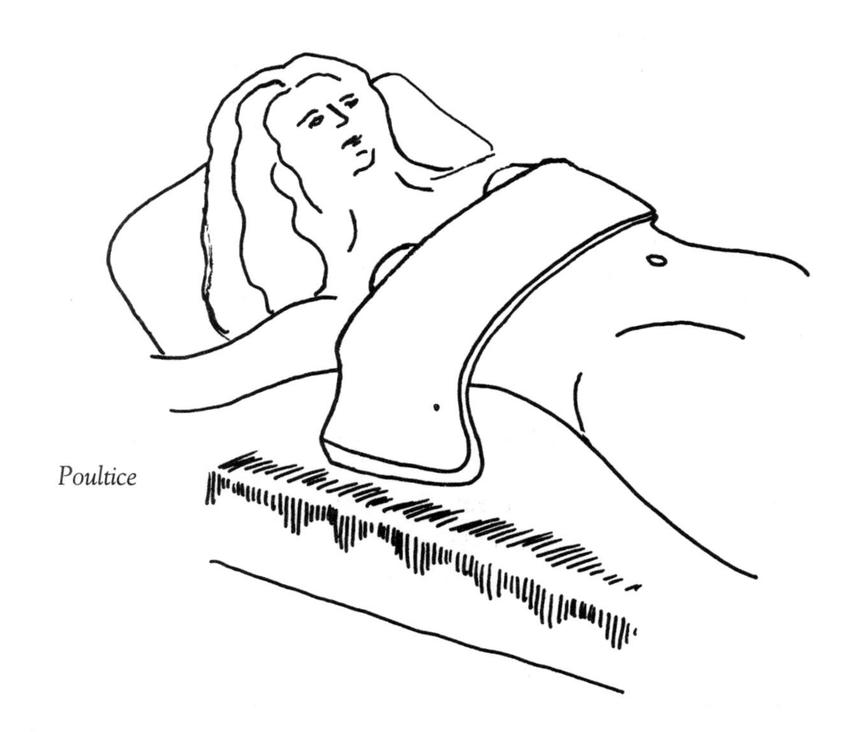

Poultice

Poultice Instructions and Supplies

1. Fresh, dried or powdered herbs; liquidized or macerated before use.

2. Slippery Elm, flour or cornstarch acts as a mucilage and holds the poultice together.

3. Honey acts as an antiseptic and anti–infectant.

4. Apple cider vinegar cleanses the skin before and after the poultices.

5. Thyme infusion is used as an antiseptic wash, especially for burns.

6. Gauze bandages or 100% fine cotton cheese cloth cut to size.

7. Saran wrap can be used to cover short–term poultices. Do not use on open wounds, burns, or when the poultice is left on all day or night, because the heat of the body causes fermentation. Chemical reactions are not good for the healing process. The skin needs to breathe and release body heat.

8. Cotton strips, stretch bandages or non–stick adhesive tape are useful to hold the poultice in place on the body.

9. A plate is required to hold the gauze bandage during the preparation process.

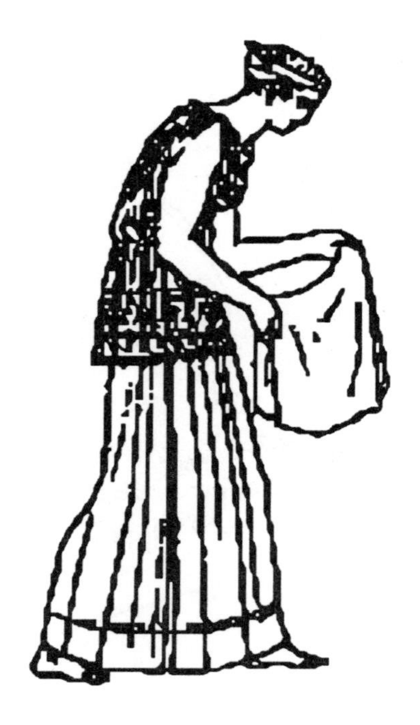

INSTRUCTIONS FOR LARGE OR SMALL POULTICES

1. Mix the selected herbs or powders together with a tablespoon or more of Slippery Elm powder, flour or cornstarch to cover the affected area well.

2. Place a gauze square on a plate, with extra material to fold over the herbs. Commercial gauze bandages open up and the herbs can be place inside, before closing again.

3. Place the herbs in the middle of the cloth. Add just enough hot water or apple cider vinegar to form a thick paste of herbs. Fold over the edges of the cloth and press out any excess moisture from the poultice. Cool to a safe temperature to suit the individual, but apply as warm as possible. Remember what is only warm to the hands feels hot to other parts of the body.

4. After bathing the area with warm apple cider vinegar or water, place the poultice over the area. Secure with stretch bandages or tape.

5. Apply the poultice in the evening and leave on all night. Moisten and reapply in the morning by turning the poultice over, or apply a new poultice. Apply a new one at night, and continue in this way until the area is healed, or instructions are changed. Short term poultices are applied for one to three hours during the day and then removed. If the area becomes tender, use a second layer of gauze and/or apply a layer of Balm of Gilead or Comfrey ointment before the poultice is applied. Make sure that the powder is finely ground to avoid irritation.

6. Moisten the poultice several times during the day with either herb teas or macerated moist herbs to prevent body heat from drying it out, especially if there is any fever. Keep it moist at all times.

7. Do not use plastic or Saran wrap unless the poultice is removed within three hours, as the excess heat and moisture will cause fermentation.

8. If the poultice sticks to an infected or raw area, begins to smell or becomes hard, soak it off in a bath of infused Thyme, Comfrey, Echinacea and Chickweed. Apply a fresh poultice. Never pull a poultice off, especially in burn cases.

Travel Poultice

Take Slippery Elm powder on camping holidays and hikes. A little water mixed with the Slippery Elm creates a gluey paste which will adhere to the skin and soothe, heal and protect wounds, bites, scratches or bruises until further treatment can be applied at home.

Prolapse Treatment

Prolapse occurs when the bowel or pelvic organs lose their tone, and the abdominal muscles lose their ability to hold the organs in place in the abdomen. This can be caused by childbirth, accidents, obesity, constipation, poor posture, aging and spinal problems. As the organs fall they cause pressure on other organs below them, and often obstruct normal functions, as well as causing pain. Prolapse of one organ or area affects all the organs in the pelvic area. Prolapse of the bowel or uterus may also cause hemorrhoids. Strengthening and astringent actions are needed to tone and contract the tissues. Body building nutrients needs to be circulated through the circulatory and lymphatic systems. The bowels must be kept active.

Infusion/ Injection Instructions

Make a concentrated infusion of the Body Building formula. Prepare one pint of the infusion by simmering two pints of distilled water mixed with four teaspoons of herb powder. Lie on a slant board, elevate the pelvis with a pillow, or hold an inverted yoga posture while retaining one quarter to one cup of the infusion in bowels. Repeat two times a day. Hold the infusion in the bowels from five to ten minutes so that the nutrient can be absorbed. In severe cases of prolapse, inject the herbal infusion into both the vagina and the rectum. It is important to drink one–quarter to three–quarters of a cup of the infusion, three times a day, or take two capsules of the powdered formula, three times a day before meals.

Inversion Therapy

Inversion therapy can be used in several different ways. Practice yoga head or shoulder stands several times daily, use slant boards, or lift the foot of the bed up at least three inches with blocks so that the prolapsed organs are relieved during the night.

Reflexology, Osteopathy & Acupuncture

Reflexology treatments increase energy to the feet and to reflex areas all over the body. Osteopathy or acupuncture stimulate the nerve supply and balance body functions, so that the maximum level of healing can be obtained. I have seen great improvements, even cures, from debilitating, weakening and painful prolapse, and since it is the sort of complaint which only gets worse if nothing is done, it is worthwhile to make efforts to regain muscular strength and tone. Use these methods along with full constitutional, eliminative and systemic care.

Poultices

My clients have achieved the best results with Comfrey and Slippery Elm abdominal poultices when they are applied together with the other treatments mentioned on this page.

Hook Treatment for Prolapse

Whenever patients suffer from prolapse I teach them a zone therapy hook technique which they practice twice a day. Regular application of these techniques definitely produces results.

1. Lie down on the bed or on the floor. Make sure the lower back and knees are supported.

2. Beginning at the eyebrows, hook all five fingers under any bone ridge, symmetrically on

both sides of the face, using both hands, and pull upward in a repetitive rhythm of five pulls. Then move down to the next bone.

3. Proceed down the body from the cheekbones, to the jawbones, the clavicles, ribs, pelvis and knees, wherever there is a bone to pull up on. In each place repeat the pull five times.

4. Repeat the cycle five times, all the while imagining that the downward prolapse tendency is being reversed and that everything is being strengthened and pulled up.

Homeopathy

The draining downward movement of prolapse is often associated with the homeopathic remedy *Sepia;* use in the 6th to 30th potency. Flower remedies are also useful to clear the mental and emotional states associated with each individual suffering from prolapse.

Referrals

Skilled practitioners of natural medicine need to learn how to refer clients for complementary treatment for the benefit of the patient. I always considered it my duty to take a course of sessions or treatments in every major form of natural medicine and experience first hand the method on my own body, as well as to read and study their therapeutic system, so that I would know when it would be appropriate to refer a patient for a specific treatment program.

Because it is too confusing to start two or more different types of treatments at once, I usually wait for a month until the picture clears with the first course of herbal treatment, diet change and naturopathic treatments before I make referrals. However, in the case of neck pain or strong symptoms, I refer clients to other practitioners immediately. Sometimes I recommend a medical test or X–ray, although most clients have usually explored this area first. It is good for patients to have further support and to experience different therapies, so that they will know in the future what will be of help to them when they have a health problem.

The School of Natural Medicine has trained many health professionals, acupuncturists, chiropractors, homeopaths, osteopaths, nurses and medical doctors, who have reported that they achieve better results when their patient completed the purification and regeneration program either before or during their treatment with them. The cleaner and clearer the body is, and the more completely the body organs, systems and glands do their work, the easier it is to respond to and maintain the improvements achieved by bodywork therapies and treatments.

Acupuncture

This is particularly useful to balance subtle meridian energies and strengthen constitutional weakness after a primary course of purification and regeneration has been completed.

Alexander Technique

This adjustment of nerves and muscles through postural alignment brings about permanent changes in the spine as well as being relaxing. My attitude toward life changed as my spine

gradually straightened during a course of Alexander sessions. I was able to communicate more clearly and directly, and I changed my life to fit my new vision. I proved the theory that lower back weakness is connected with lack of will and strength on mental and emotional levels. Two years of Alexander sessions in Cambridge, England, straightened my spine which had always been curved by a congenital sway–back condition. As well as giving me a new outlook on life, I saved a small fortune in chiropractic and osteopathic adjustments. For many years I have used the exercises the practitioner taught me to self–adjust my spine. These exercises when combined with baths, reflexology and self–massage successfully enable me to avoid having to have regular spinal adjustments. However, when osteopathic and chiropractic adjustments are necessary, I don't hesitate. Every system of healing has its place. If adjustments aren't working, try the Alexander technique.

Chiropractic and Osteopathy

Whenever the iris reveals structural weakness, toxins or inflammation in spinal and neck areas or whenever there is pain, support any natural medicine internal treatment by having spinal and cranial/sacral adjustments. For those who are having regular adjustments, they will find that the treatments will hold better, and that the muscles return to health more quickly, when the body is supported by internal herbal treatment and improved diet. Do not become dependent on regular adjustments.

Massage and Body Work

Any form of bodywork that relaxes, releases tension and tones the body, as well as deeper body work that brings to the surface somatic emotions and uncompleted memories, supports the self healing process. Excellent body–centered therapies are rolfing, rosen work, hakomi, reiki, neuromuscular massage, shiatsu, jin jin jitsu, trager work, or deep tissue massage. Build a network of practitioners to support any health difficulties.

Polarity Therapy

Polarity sessions offer a deep balancing of the elements of life that brings emotions up to the surface and creates harmonious patterns. Polarity is especially recommended when there is a strong excess or shortage of any emotion.

Reflexology

I highly recommend this foot reflex massage therapy. It is a valuable for clients to learn how to apply it themselves, as well as to receive treatments to augment any purification or healing program. It is important to give each client every possible tool to apply at home. Not only does this speed the healing process, but it helps people to get in touch with their own body and to explore the world of natural and alternative healing.

For years I had a small practice at home when my children were growing up. During the consultation I soaked clients' feet in herbal brews while I took their case history and read their eyes. I then gave them a thorough reflexology treatment, which always confirmed what the iris revealed about their inner condition. I taught them how to work on their reflexology points at home to speed progress and to inspire them to develop skills to help make them independently healthy.

Skin Care

Skin is more than just a body wrapping; it is the largest organ of the body. Good health depends on the skin performing its two–fold duties of respiration and excretion. If it is not performing these duties, the kidneys, liver, lungs and lymph have to compensate. Skin problems can also be the result of poorly functioning eliminative organs, particularly the kidneys, the bowels and the liver.

Skin inactivity is due to several causes, or a combination of them, from poor and irregular bathing habits, to the wearing of synthetic fabrics and lack of exercise. Jethro Kloss, in his natural health book *Back to Eden*, claims that inactivity of the skin is one of the main causes of all skin diseases, combined with poor eating habits, and that any person who wishes to cure any physical problem, or to enjoy an excellent standard of health, must apply therapeutic means to establish normal skin function.

Our skin is an organ of respiration and excretion. It absorbs oxygen and water and exhales poisonous gases. The skin also absorbs whatever lotions, creams or oils we use on our skin or in our baths. We should never use anything on the skin that we would not eat, as our body must assimilate, metabolize and eliminate anything we apply on it. Mineral oil cannot be absorbed. It clogs the pores, and draws B vitamins from the body. Pure vegetable oils or natural organic creams are not only readily absorbed by the body but also contribute to positive improvement by feeding the skin and providing the necessary moisture and nourishment for suppleness and skin tone.

The skin has millions of pores from which a constant stream of acids and toxins flow. If these pores are blocked, the toxins collect in the skin and lymph, or return to the liver, forcing extra work on an active major organ. Bathing and brushing the skin is important, so that dead dry skin is shed, allowing fresh skin to breathe and eliminate without inhibition. Hot and cold alternating temperatures in bathing, showering, saunas and packs exercise the skin, and increase and equalize the circulation, so that each part of the body receives its equal share of life–giving blood. Cold water contracts the blood vessels and lessens the amount of blood at the surface. Hot water draws the blood back to the surface, stimulating and giving relief to the organs under the skin as it breaks up congestion. Cold water alkalinizes the blood. That is one of the reasons we feel refreshed and bright after cool sprays and dips following hot showers or baths.

Good bathing and cleansing habits are essential for good health. We have heard it said that cleanliness is next to Godliness. Prophets and yogis guide their followers to be scrupulously clean. Plants appear fresher and brighter after a shower, and birds and animals do not neglect their daily wash. Similarly for us, daily baths and showers are ideal. When skin pores open during baths, toxins are eliminated.

The skin also regulates the body temperature. Usually it prevents the escape of body heat, but during fevers, exercise and heat, the skin sweats and lets the heat escape. The regular intake of pure water together with sponging the body aids this process. When water surrounds the body it influences the nervous system through the skin because the skin has nerve receptors which are closely connected with all the major nerve plexuses. The skin also helps us by storing large quantities of water and salts, resisting the invasion of germs and absorbing gases and fatty substances. It is richly supplied with blood vessels. The sebaceous glands in the skin secrete a greasy substance which keeps the skin soft and supple.

VAGINAL AND PROSTATE OVULE TREATMENT

Vaginal Ovule

Combine the vaginal ovule formula powder with an equal amount of Slippery Elm powder. Mix well by shaking both together in a plastic bag.

Buy coconut oil or coconut butter from a health food store or delicatessen. Soften it over a very low heat. Add in one drop of Tea Tree oil. Mix the oil with the powder until you obtain a doughy paste. When the oil hardens the ovules in the fridge it will hold the powder in shape. The best method for rolling the ovule shape is to place the mixture on a small, plastic sandwich baggie and shape into a long tube. The baggie keeps your hands clean and gives a smooth finish. Cut the tube into one inch lengths. Lift the ovules while still on the plastic bag and place them in the refrigerator to harden. Wrap them inside the baggie.

Each day that you use the ovules, put in one or two of the one–inch length ovules, depending on the size of the vagina and the severity of the condition. The average program is one of the one–inch length ovules. If you want a strong program, it is easier to push in three short one–inch ovules one after another than trying to push in a three–inch long one.

I have experienced a wide variety of responses from women, all the way from: “I put it in and it disappears. Where does it go?” to “It falls out all the time. I can’t keep it in.” Many women find that the ovules stay relatively solid and come out easily using either a finger or the douches. They also find they need to hold the vagina closed so that the ovule will stay in place when they are pressing down muscles for bowel movements.

It is helpful to plug the opening of the vagina with cotton batten, a homemade tampon of natural sea sponge, or an end cut from a tampon. You can press on the tampon so that it won’t come out during bowel movements. Most women dread this treatment unnecessarily, thinking that it will be difficult and messy. Following the instructions keeps mess to the minimum, and the results are well worth the effort.

It is best to prepare a week’s supply of ovules at one time and keep them ready in the refrigerator. Since a fresh supply is needed twice a day five times a week, ten or more ovules are required per week, or an adjusted number according to the condition and the size of the vagina.

We advise wearing black underpants during this treatment, so that they are not ruined by stains. Some women may also need to wear a mini–pad. Experiment and adjust the treatment to specific needs, so that it is comfortable and easy to do it.

Although we recommend abstaining from sexual intercourse during the vaginal treatment, if partners cannot wait to make love, do so after removing the ovule and douching with Yellow Dock. Douche again after making love, then continue the program.

Prostate Ovule

Add one ounce of the Prostate herbal formula to the ovule mix. Insert ovules into the rectum after each bowel movement, using one or two, one–inch ovules daily. Following the treatment schedule on the next page, retain the herbal rectal injection for five to ten minutes after the bowel has been washed clean with a water enema. Use Castor oil packs before, during and after the prostate ovule treatment. Take bowel herbs. It is beneficial to have an iridology analysis. Take the full constitutional treatment program to overcome prostate weakness.

Treatment Schedule for Vaginal or Prostate Ovule

Monday a.m.

Insert one to three one–inch ovules into the vagina or rectum. Leave them in all day. Hold in place with a sponge or cut tampon. Replace it if it comes out. Insert a fresh ovule and leave it in all night. Insert a new ovule on Tuesday morning after moving the bowels. Use an enema if necessary before inserting the prostate ovule in the rectum.

Tuesday p.m.

Douche the vagina or rectum with one cup of well strained Yellow Dock or Burdock infusion. Inject the cup while you are in an inverted position. Lifting the pelvis up, or using pillows to hold the pelvis up. Retain the fluid inside the vagina or rectum at least five minutes so that it can be absorbed into the mucus membranes, tissues, blood and lymph. Visualize that the ovules are spreading their positive influence into the pelvis. Lie in the bath to keep warm and relaxed. Douche with Thyme tea or Tea Tree oil if there are Candida Albicans or thrush problems. Take an enema before the prostate ovule. Insert another ovule into the vagina or rectum. Leave in overnight until Wednesday morning.

Wednesday, Thursday and Friday

Repeat the Monday and Tuesday procedures until Saturday.

Saturday p.m.

Remove the ovule, douche, but do not insert another ovule until Monday morning, when the entire procedure is repeated for up to a period of seven weeks, then have a break. Many patients report that not much happens until the third or fourth week. Discharges, odors and other reactions are normal as toxins and mucus are released. Support the treatment with internal herbs and a purification diet.

If possible, women should continue the ovule treatment throughout their monthly menstrual cycle. When the flow is heavy, count off the days of strong flow and resume the same weekly schedule when the flow is light enough. You may need to replace the ovule more often, or use it just at night

Follow Up

When you wish to take a rest from the full vaginal ovule treatment, continue the impetus of purification by douching with Yellow Dock tea or Thyme tea at regular intervals according to need.

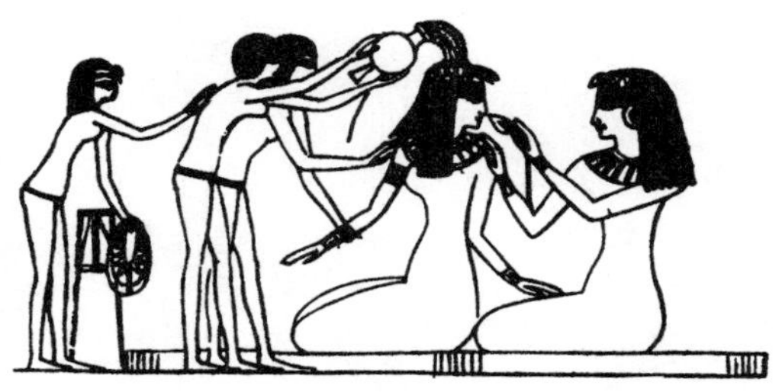

7

Iridology & Inner Ecology

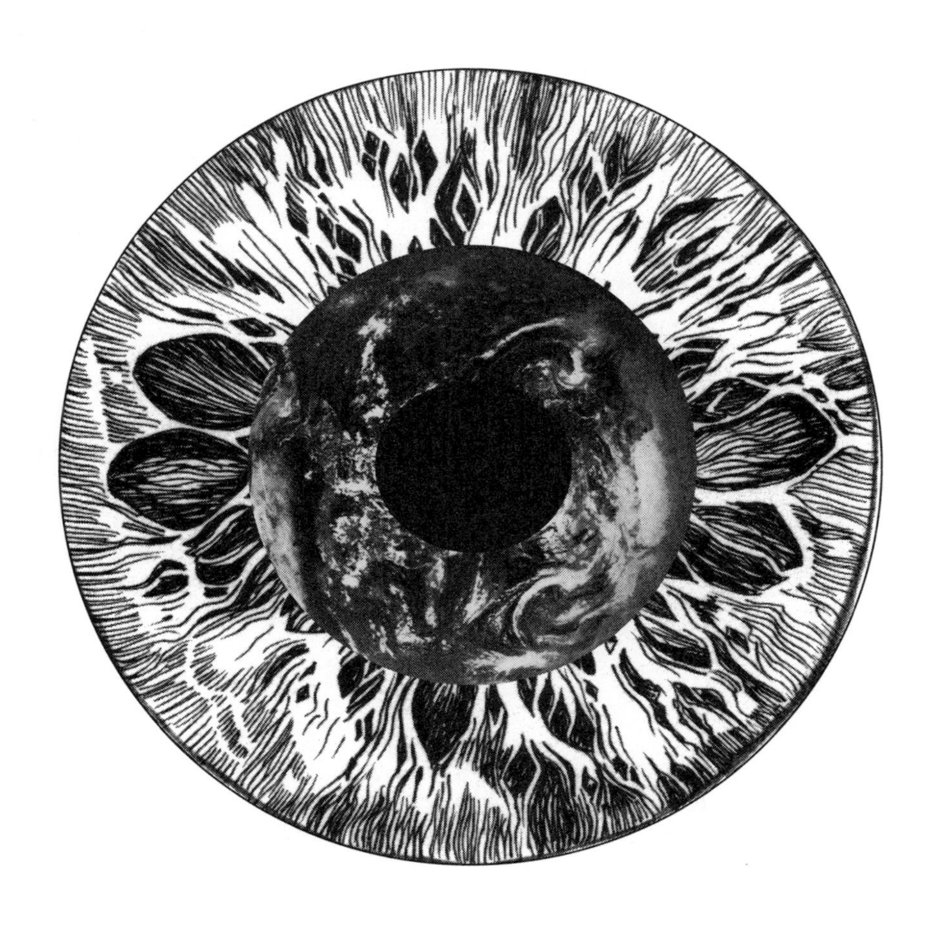

Iridology & Inner Ecology

THE EYES OF THE WORLD

All living creatures have eyes that look into the world and share the spirit of life with each other's eyes. Whenever we meet the living eyes of any species, we can feel their spirit and their life. There is an exchange of energy and a connection is established.

The pupil reveals the eyelight of the spirit. The iris, the colored area that surrounds the pupil, is a mirror of the inner world, the only original brain tissue to meet the outside world.

Connected through the hypothalamus, the irides reveal information about the condition of all parts of the body in all dimensions of being, body, emotions, mind and spirit. Many of the mysteries and beauties of life are revealed there, but we can only receive the information according to the level of our consciousness. Learning to see the connectedness of life, both inwardly through iridology and outwardly in the world, is a state of grace that grows out of respect and love. The iris becomes our teacher when we look at it under magnification because it gives us new information. The holographic iris reveals the fullness of all aspects of our being.

When we learn about iridology, we begin to see in a holistic, ecological way, and we open to the relationships between our organs, systems and glands, our emotions, our mental patterns and our karmic destiny. We also begin to understand how our inner ecology affects and influences the outer ecology of our world. Our mind expands and evolves. It becomes more fluid, less judgmental and more open to change and tolerance. It learns to see in all directions at once. Our vision opens to a wide horizon of possibilities all related by connectedness – the essence of ecology. Iridology and ecology blend into each other and become iricology.

IRIS COLORS

There are two iris colors, brown and blue, and all other colors display themselves against this background or change the appearance of the background by a anotehr layer of color; yellow covering blue makes a greenish color, for example. There are many different shades of brown and blue, and a third mixed type, displays both colors. Other colors such as orange, yellow, rust, cream or white in many different shades are the result of body chemistry, digestive processes, environmental pollution, food additives, preservatives, aging and medication. Some of these colors are inherited, some develop during our lives, and some change during purification treatment. The significance of the most important colors are explained during a personal iris analysis. If you have a deeper interest I recommend purchasing my book *Iridology – a complete guide to iris analysis*, published by Thorsons division of HarperCollins, now out of print. Copies can be purchased from the School of Natural Medicine. Wisdome Press is republishing *Iridology* in spring 1995. Iridology correspondence courses and seminars are also available. See the application form at the back of the book for prices, information and a free brochure.

Inner Ecology Reflects Outer Ecology

Iridology also shows us that inner ecology reflects outer ecology, and outer ecology reflects inner ecology. From the viewpoint of this perception we can say that our diseased and unbalanced inner world is a reflection of the diseased and unbalanced outer world, or the reverse. This ecological relationship of excesses and shortages, stresses and strains, weaknesses and strengths, must be balanced and healed within us, so that the world we live in can be healed and balanced by our positive influence. Greater harmony between inner and outer world reduces stress and creates a life of ease, peace and contentment.

In this stressful material world most people live their lives in relationship to the outer world, never realizing how important it is to build up a relationship with the inner life so that the forces from the world are met with strength and balance from within. This balance enables us to build an inner reality which positively influences the world and allows us to rejuvenate and nourish ourselves. Healing becomes a way of life that is lived moment to moment because we are in touch with the essence of our own reality and are not driven entirely by the demands of the outside world.

The world within our body reflects the same natural principles as our outer world. Both are based on ecological laws of homeostasis or balance and of shortage or excess when out of balance. Just as a shortage of water produces a drought and an excess, floods, lack of feeling produces dryness or apathy, and excess, hysteria and passion. The dance of the elements within and without our body creates the climate of our holographic life. Both our inner world of physical organs, systems and glands, and our interaction with the world as we take in or release physically, emotionally, mentally and spiritually, are revealed in the irides

Inner Ecology, Iridology & Iricology

Iridology means the study of the iris of the eye. Ecology means the study of the relationships between living organisms and their environment (both inner and outer). Iricology is the holistic ecological study of the microcosm of the inner world and the macrocosm of the outer world in relationship, as observed in the iris of the eye. Iridology is a doorway to our inner ecology, the fundamental inherited inter–relationship of our organs, systems and glands which reveal the pathways to personality, aging and the development of acute and chronic illness.

The iris of the eye displays life processes, energies and movements against the constitutional fabric of life. It is best if this information is received when we are young, so that we have the opportunity for prevention through conscious life choices that do not aggravate and accelerate our inherent weaknesses. Our weaknesses are only potential. Whatever seeds we sow, whether they be for health or illness, will develop in our constitutional soil.

Because iridology also offers information about our strengths, our personality and our potential, there is much to learn from an analysis. Our entire being, body, mind, emotions and spirit is revealed in our irides if we have the eyes to see and the openness to receive.

Healing requires truth and a deep level of holistic perception and education. The ancient naturopaths in Greece put the words 'Know Thyself' above their doorways. Our eyes are the threshold to our inner world, and we can use the information they give us to guide us in that exploration. If we truly did know ourselves we would have the answer as to why we needed an illness, and we would know what we had to do. This journey to 'knowing ourself and healing ourself' is our true path. I wish you joy and success on your journey.

Iris Fiber Structure – The Fabric of Life

Iris fibers, when fine and tightly woven, represent structural strength. Loose fibers display open emotional receptivity, release and expression. Both are valuable qualities. Strong examples of one type or another show that the missing aspect needs to be developed for balance. A type that has all aspects in an average balance reveals another kind of strength, that of openness and understanding for others and an ability to access visual, auditory and kinesthetic modes of learning and expression. The different types of iris structures are displayed below: Silk, Cotton, Linen, Muslin, Burlap, and Zig Zag.

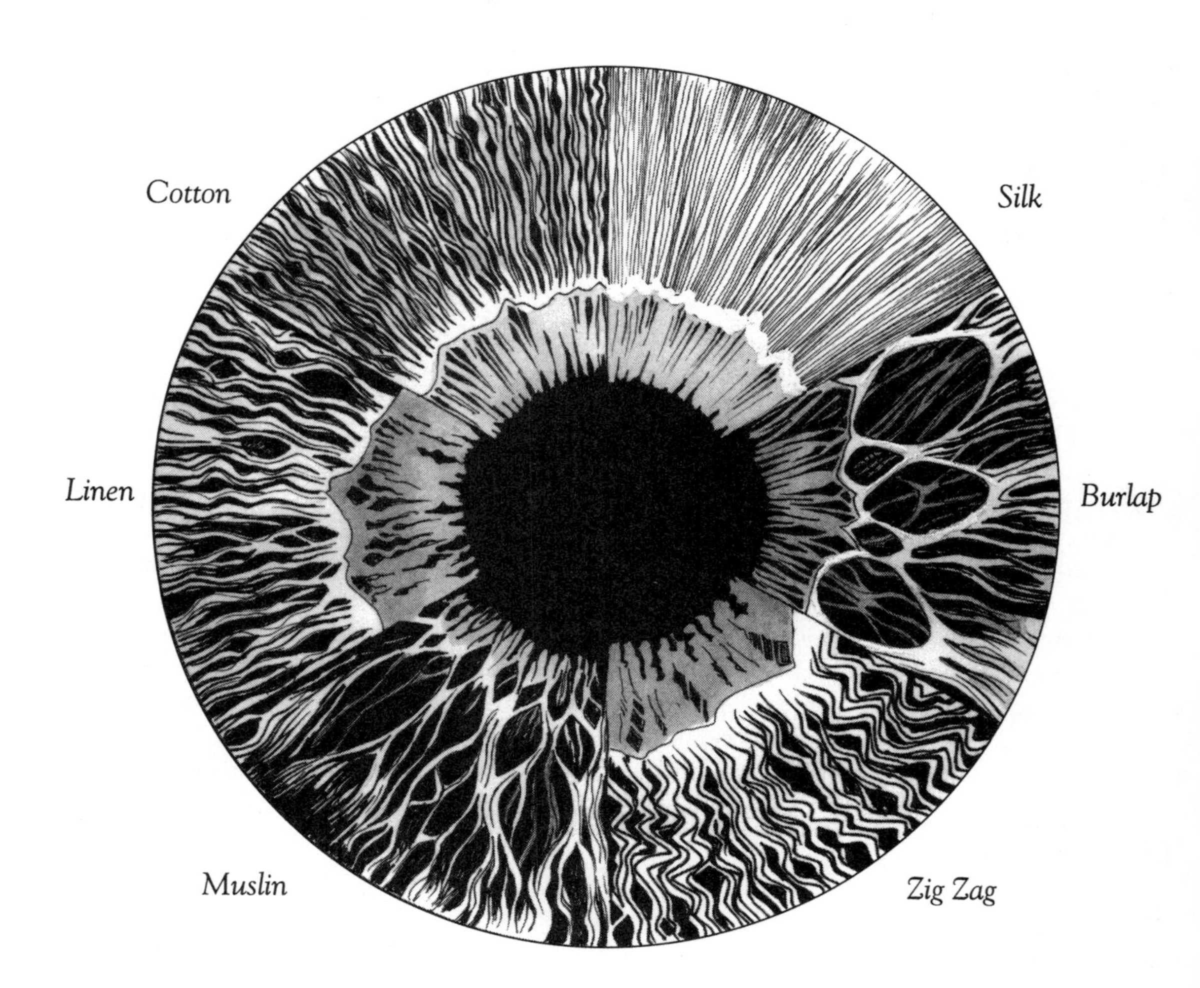

Iris Structural Types

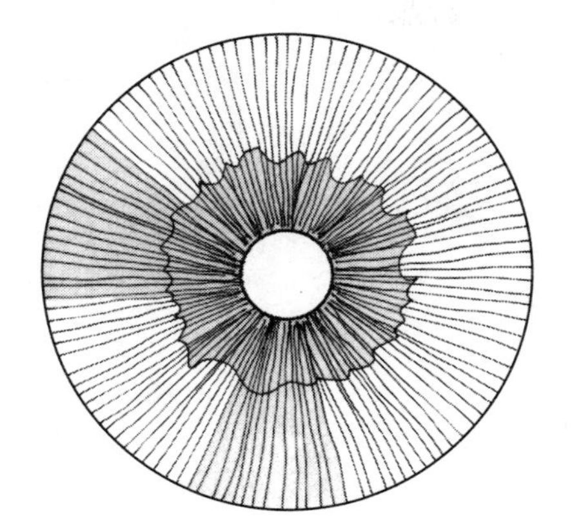

Silk Structure Type – Pioneer Activist Person

Positive Aspects – a strong structure with a quick recuperative ability, energetic goal achievers who can work long hours without rest or sleep, and natural leaders and visionaries who express verbally and learn visually; because they are such a strong type, they often attract and marry their opposite, someone emotional and expressive, for balance.

Negative Aspects – intolerant of others who are weaker or who have less energy, they drive their body to the breaking point as they dominate and manipulate others to achieve their goals; they have difficulty coming out of their head into their feelings, and expressing emotions.

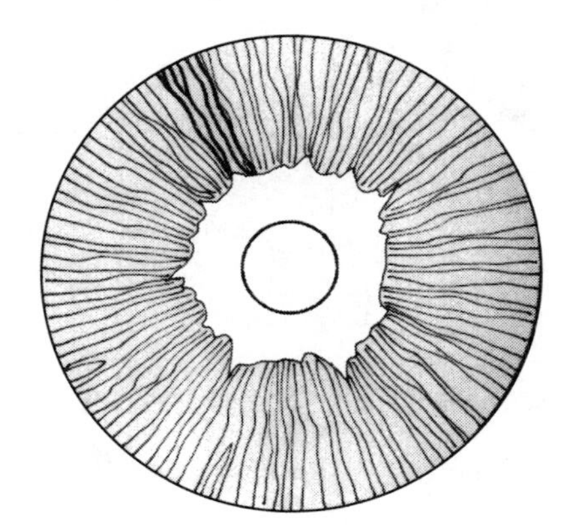

Linen Structure Type – Strong Worker Person

Positive Aspects – they have a good measure of the Silk positive qualities, including strong energy and health, with more access to feeling, expression and sensitivity to others.

Negative Aspects – they are less rigid than the negative Silk type; they are beginning to appreciate leisure and the value of '*being*' instead of always working on goal oriented projects.

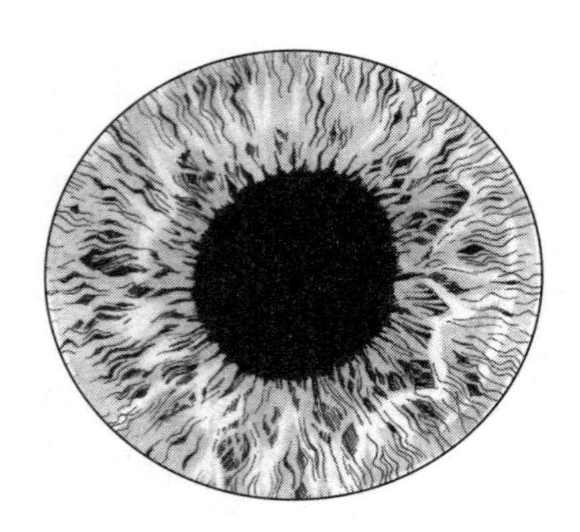

COTTON STRUCTURE TYPE – AVERAGE COMFORTABLE PERSON

Positive Aspects – their strength manifests through balance and a more expressive emotional life; they enjoy all aspects of life: work, sociability, solitude and leisure; they are less obsessive than Silk or Linen and more structured than the Burlap type.

Negative Aspects – they can be without strong focus or try to go in too many directions because many avenues are open to them; they rely on what is easy, rather than make effort, and may lack purpose because their nature is not strong in any direction; they may settle for a situation below their capability just to make life easy.

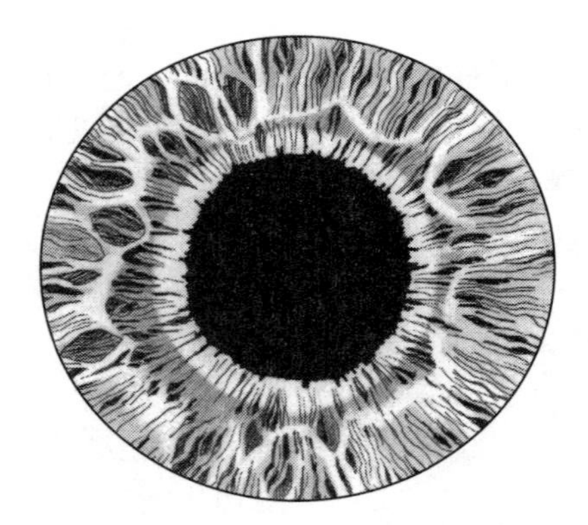

MUSLIN STRUCTURE TYPE – FEELING CREATIVE PERSON

Positive Aspects – empathetic, creative and expressive individuals with sensitive, strong instincts and feelings, they can release and communicate through voice, writing, dance, art, poetry and color; they adjust to circumstances easily and have compassion for those around them as well as concern for the environment.

Negative Aspects – they can be overly emotional, lack structure, and be gifted but unable to organize themselves to achieve goals; they live in the realm of ideas rather than manifesting their visions, and can get lost in dreams, fantasies and projections; they are weaker physically, with slow recuperative abilities, need more rest, and are affected easily by others; they have long range stamina for survival.

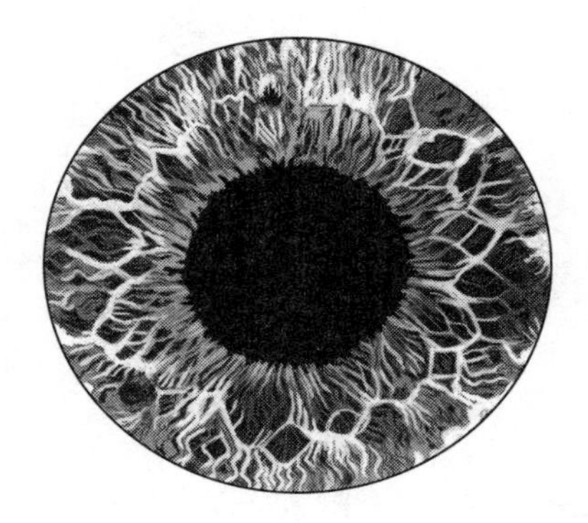

BURLAP STRUCTURE TYPE – SURVIVOR ADJUSTER PERSON

Positive Aspects – they have an increased capacity for tolerance, understanding and compassion in difficult circumstances, letting events and difficulties flow around and through them rather than holding on and creating resistance or reactions; they offer leadership based on feeling the needs of others, rather than pushing everyone to achieve a goal regardless of individual sacrifices.

Negative Aspects – they suffer from weak recuperative ability, low energy, low resistance to disease, digestive and structural weakness, and apathy.

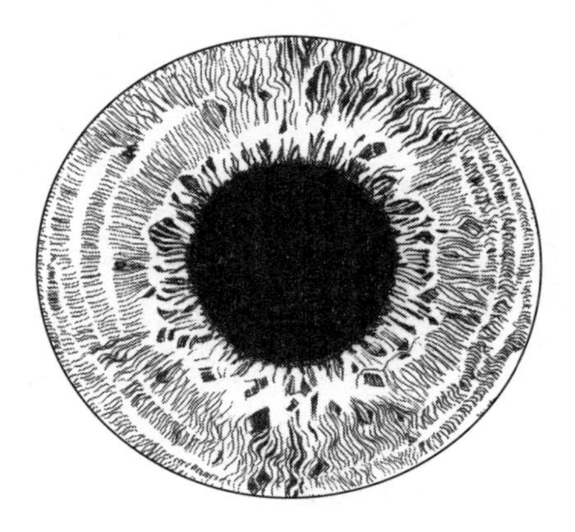

ZIG ZAG STRUCTURE TYPE – NERVOUS CONFLICT PERSON

Positive Aspects – their increased sensitivity gives them the ability to look at different sides of any situation.

Negative Aspects – because of indecision they experience an inability to move ahead without chopping and changing; this difficulty in achieving goals leads to hypersensitivity, impatience and exhaustion due to the mental conflict; it is important that this type should not stay in a situation they cannot resolve.

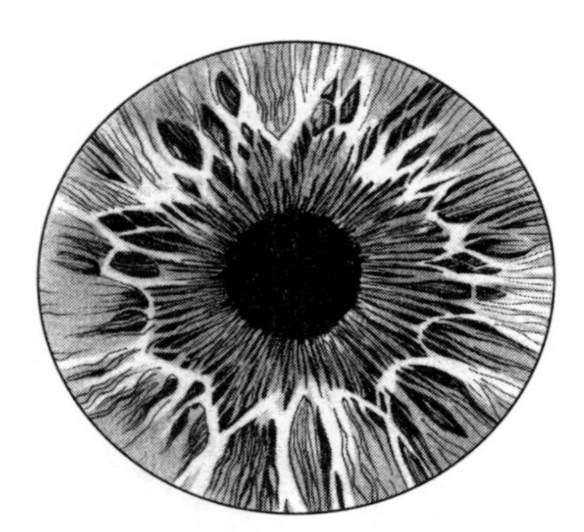

Net Structure Type – Creates Own Reality Person

Positive Aspects – this type creates a net effect that rises up on the surface of the iris, usually a white upper layer with darker tones in the lower layer; the net filters difficult experiences; they have the strength of the net combined with endurance, cheeriness and enthusiastic optimism.

Negative Aspects – their weakness lies in not facing things as they are; they fantasize or select, leaving out much; they often do not face the negative side of life, preferring to live in their own reality, according to their dream vision; often childlike, they can avoid responsibilities and duties; physically, the autonomic nervous system can become exhausted, and deep toxins can collect beneath any overactive net fibers; the polarities of life are so separated that the iris shows two levels; eventually the polarities meet when the body breaks down and reality must be faced.

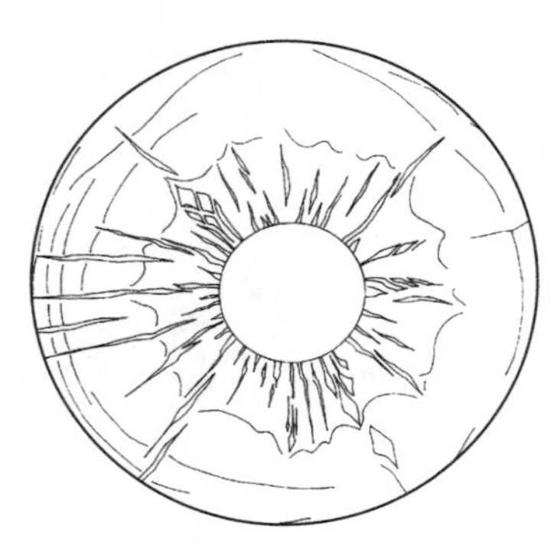

Velvet Non-Structure Type – Silent Pathology Person

Positive Aspects – true brown eyes do not reveal iris fibers and do not have a structural pattern; this lack of reactivity on the surface creates the ability to live without distractions, and to plod on, day by day, without much thought for the body or self; this approach to life benefits family and community; the individual takes care of their body and appreciates preventive care and reasonable living habits.

Negative Aspects – the ability to ignore the body and not take care of it until something chronic manifests is a problem with this type; they need to get in touch with, receive and respond to body messages of stress or malfunction; read the Velvet Brown constitutional type to learn more.

IRIDOLOGY CONSTITUTIONS

Certain combinations of body systems appear together in the iris and create patterns which are organized into constitutional types. Each type reveals a combination of sensitivity and weakness. Their constititional selection of organs, systems and glands weaves the fabric of each person's inherent body/mind/spirit dynamic. Imbalances in any organ, system or gland affects the function of other organs, systems and glands, which then must adjust and compensate. When we approach healing with this deep level of information we can activate, support, rejuvenate and balance systemic function, so that optimum levels of health, healing and energy can be achieved.

The constitutional fabric of life, the iris structure, depicts the potential life story. Knowing the gifts and limitations of our type helps us to develop our strengths, and strengthen our weaknesses. Otherwise we are at the mercy of ignorance, a victim of our body reality. This information is not something to be feared. It is not a judgment. It tells us more of who and what we are and what we have to work with. It is enlightenment. The purpose of this work is not only to help prevent the development of constitutional aging illness but to restore health that has been lost through ignorance, stress, overwork and carelessness.

Certain iris patterns appear again and again, and when we correlate symptoms, aging processes, diseases and personality tendencies, distinct types emerge. The patterns help us to understand the causes of our imbalances and illnesses. We learn that we are not alone in the way our body is aging or developing disease. We learn that there are reasons for the health problems that we have, and we learn what we can do about it.

There is no good constitution, nor is there a bad constitution. Each constitution has its strengths and weaknesses. Because each constitution involves not only the physical reality but the emotions, mind and spirit, extreme strength in one aspect does not necessarily mean strength in them all. Strong structural types are often emotionally insensitive and unable to enjoy life when they are not in full drive, achieving goals; therefore their weakness is in the emotional life.

Some individuals display strong types and others are a mixture of two, three or more types. Just because you are a certain constitutional type or types does not mean that you will develop the common conditions which persons of this type or types are prone to develop. These conditions are potential only. They reveal the inherent pathways of aging and chronic illness that are activated by how we live in our body. This system is used for educational purposes, not for the diagnosis of disease.

It is also important to remember that the constitutional types are a description of the main background patterns against which all other colors, openings, lines and markings on the iris display themselves in a more complex, uniquely individual way. The full picture is explained in an individual iridology analysis. Models of each of the main systemic constitutional types are included here as an individual educational reference.

Some of the information listed under a type may be relevant and some may not. It is essential for people interested in their own health and well–being to have an iris analysis for self education. This work does not replace professional medical advice, diagnosis or treatment.

Immune Reactive

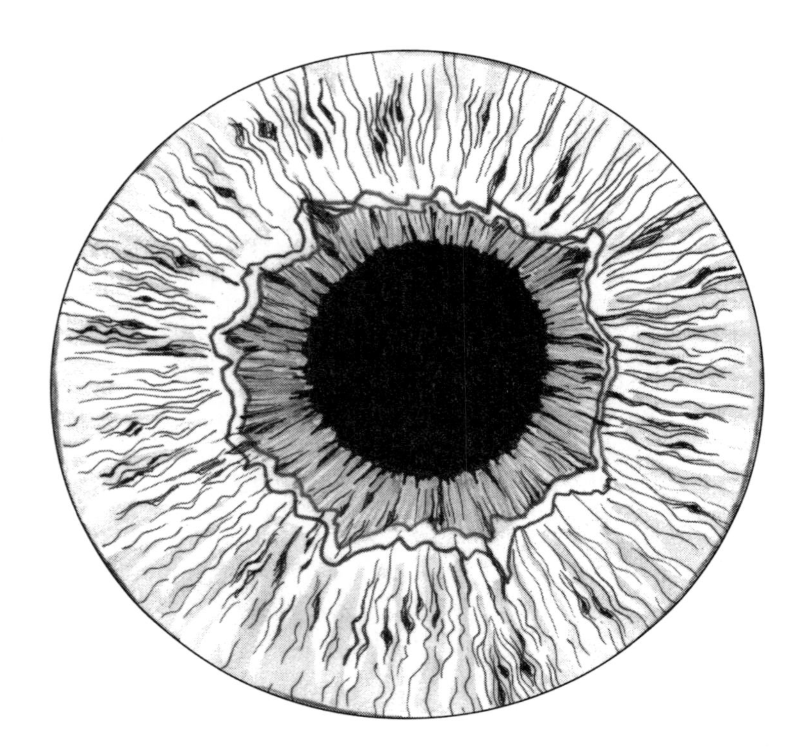

Iris Color	Blue
Fiber Structure	Average
Description	Raised thick, often swollen collarette or nerve wreath
Aging/Disease Pathways	Lymphatic system reactivity related to the autonomic nervous system
Systems	Lymphatic, nervous
Other Possible Signs	White autonomic nerve collarette; white lymph zones where the ear, nose, eyes, vagina or rectum open to the outside world; white fiber strands moving out from the digestive areas into the iris

Tissue Weakness	Mucus membranes, lymph glands, eliminative discharges through nasal and gastrointestinal tract, sense organs, reproductive organs
Gland Weakness	Lymph glands
Organ Weakness	None unless other iris signs denote them
Activity	Acute discharges, hyperactive and chronic inflammation, constant internal energetic aggression against the environment and invaders
Symptoms	Acne, aching muscles, adenoids, allergies, arthritis, coughs, dandruff, dry skin, eczema, eye irritations and discharges, nasal congestion, sinus, sneezing, stiffness, swollen glands, vaginal discharges, water retention
Eliminate	Dairy, acid or mucus forming foods, sugar, alcohol
Diet	Mucus–free diet, alkaline foods, sufficient fluids
Lifestyle	Regular exercise, reduced contact with environmental and dietary pollutants, must develop moderation and discrimination
Herbs	Lymphatic, Antibiotics Naturally, Infection, Mucus Congestion, Chronic Purifier formulae
Treatments	Glandular poultices

Personality

The hyperactive response of this type is created by overenthusiasm and reactivity. They are tuned into and touched by everything. The constant stimulation creates restlessness which causes further reactivity and chemistry imbalances. This results in continuous discharges and acute symptoms which are a continual source of low–grade infection and stress. This further weakens the body. When this type learns strength and stillness in their inner world so that the outer world does not overstimulate them, together with appropriate diet and living habits, their sensitivity can be utilized without it being a constant source of stress and irritation. Over time they will develop a sense of ease in relationship to the world. Their membrane of reaction between the inner and outer worlds is very thin so that great care needs to be taken in the maturing process to work with this sensitivity, rather than become its victim.

Challenge

Avoid the suppression of symptoms and the development of chronic disease by calming and neutralizing reactivity. It is important that the body and life are not always in a state of defense, insecurity, hyperactivity and reactivity. Keep the immune system clean and clear and support it during reactivity and acute conditions.

Nervous Sensitive

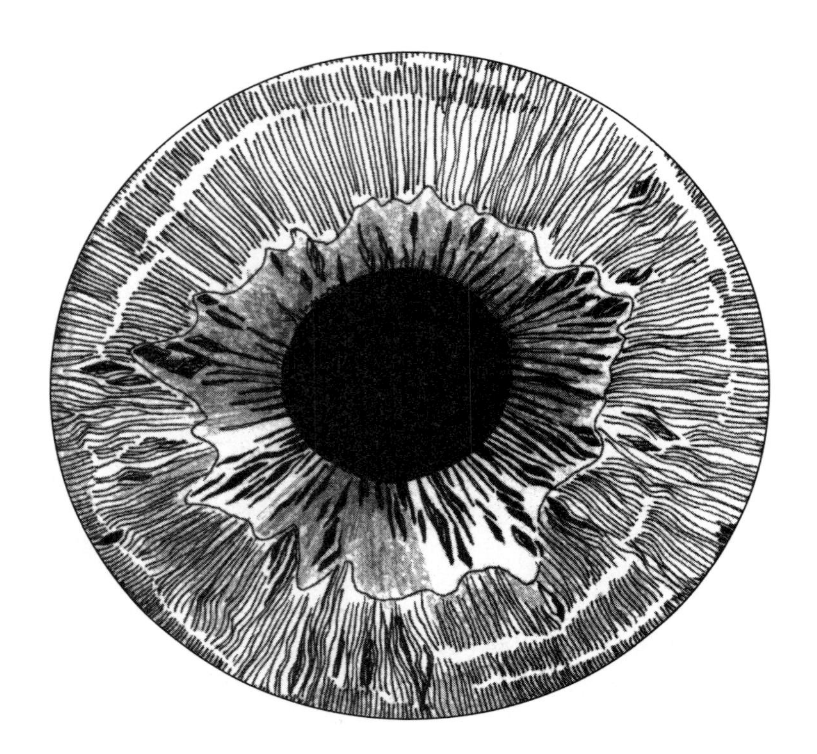

Iris Color	Blue
Fiber Structure	Linen; fine, wiry fibers
Description	Strong to average structure with a white collarette
Aging/Disease Pathways	Nervous system
Systems	Nervous, endocrine, muscular
Other Possible Signs	Glandular weakness, white fibers, skin toxicity, hyperactive brain areas; inflammatory processes are the result of nerve sensitivity and depletion; sensitivity rings or other nerve signs displayed over this background indicate stronger sensitivity

Tissue Weakness	Nerves, skin, muscles, brain tissues
Gland Weakness	Adrenals, thyroid
Organ Weakness	None unless depicted by other signs
Activity	Inflammation, thyroid–related calcium imbalances, nerve irritation and sensitivity
Symptoms	Arthritis, calcium deficiency or excess, headaches, hypersensitivity, migraines, nerve afflictions such as shingles and multiple sclerosis, skin eruptions, ulcers, vascular spasms
Eliminate	Stimulants, stress, overwork
Diet	Alkaline, calming foods; avoid overeating or eating late at night
Lifestyle	Moderation and balance; learn relaxation; take regular breaks and adequate sleep to restore the nervous system
Herbs	Adrenal, Calcium, Nerve, Thyroid, Sweet Sleep formulae
Treatments	Castor oil packs on the solar plexus, energy balancing bodywork, grounding exercises; acupuncture; massage

Personality

These are success–oriented people who can blind themselves to what is around them due to limited goal vision. They sacrifice too much to achieve their goals and get what they want. Ultimately their overdrive results in burnout, exhaustion, collapse, strokes or chronic disease. Adjustment to a restricted lifestyle is very difficult. Their structural strength gives them the energy to achieve goals and work hard, but when the use of stimulants and stressful lifestyles put them in hyper–drive, they deplete their adrenals and nervous system. Their air element imbalance creates speed and greed which further stresses the limited vision of goal pressures.

Challenge

They need to learn 'to be' instead of always 'to do,' to become human beings instead of human doings. Vision must open to include all of life, not just goals. It is also important for this type to learn tolerance for others who are different.

Lymphatic Sensitive

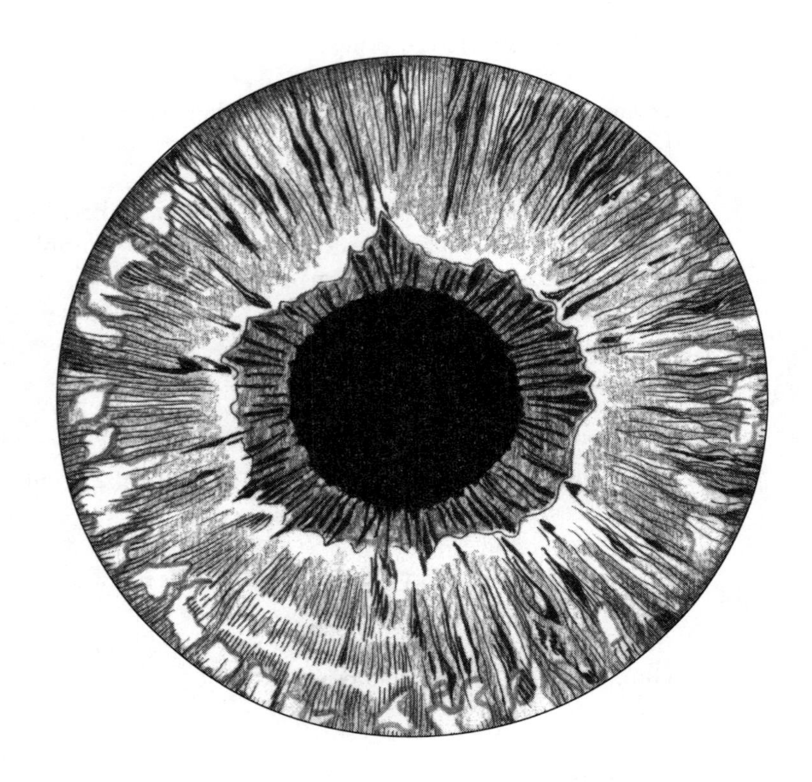

Iris Color	Blue
Fiber Structure	Any structure
Description	Partial or complete circular peripheral lymphatic tophi
Aging/Disease Pathways	Lymphatic system
System	Lymphatic
Other Possible Signs	Varying colors of white, grey, yellow or brown lymphatic tophi in areas around and within the ciliary outer iris edge; whitening of the iris fibers; often combined with dense, deep sensitivity rings; gray extends into sclera at 9 and 3 o'clock, on one or both eyes, lateral or medial

Tissue Weakness	All body tissues are affected by lymphatic malfunction
Gland Weakness	None unless depicted by lacunae or radii soleris
Organ Weakness	Spleen or any other organ depicted by lacunae or radii soleris
Activity	Imbalances in lymphatic function, tissue fluid imbalances, inflammation, hyperactive or hypoactive immunity
Symptoms	Acute discharges, allergies, hay fever, edema, rheumatism, swollen glands
Eliminate	Dairy foods, mucus forming foods, sugar, processed foods and acid foods; avoid meat and alcohol
Diet	Natural whole foods, organic raw and cooked fruits and vegetables, grains, nuts, seeds, vegetable juices, adequate liquid intake daily
Lifestyle	Regular exercise, avoid smog, pollution, car fumes; avoid contaminants from paint, preservatives, chemicals and hair and beauty products
Herbs	Lymphatic, Blood Purifying, Chronic Purifier and Circulation formulae; drink Fenugreek tea (6 to 8 c daily) or take powder in capsules
Treatments	Poultices, aerobic exercise, lymph massage, regular walking, beauty, music

Personality

This personality reflects the quality of the lymphatic system. They have ideals of harmony, peace and purity, a heaven on earth idealistic vision. They feel kinesthetically the suffering of other living beings, the decimation of wildlife, and the pollution of the planet. They work tirelessly for causes and have difficulty saying no. When they become depressed they wallow in emotional toxicity. Harmonious beauty, music, art or literature lifts their spirits and inspires them. Because they are greatly affected by the environment, they need to surround themselves with beauty and harmony, especially in the home and work environment.

Challenge

Because the tendency of this type is to hold on to toxicity, it is essential that efforts be made to learn to release, to let go and purify on all levels. Whenever this type holds on to toxins or unexpressed emotions, the lymph becomes congested and affects the entire body. The nature of lymph is to flow, to purify and to circulate throughout the entire body, restoring balance, harmony and purity throughout the tissues. It is also essential that this type learns to say no, not to overload their systems, and to discriminate carefully as to what they allow into their life.

Lymphatic Holding

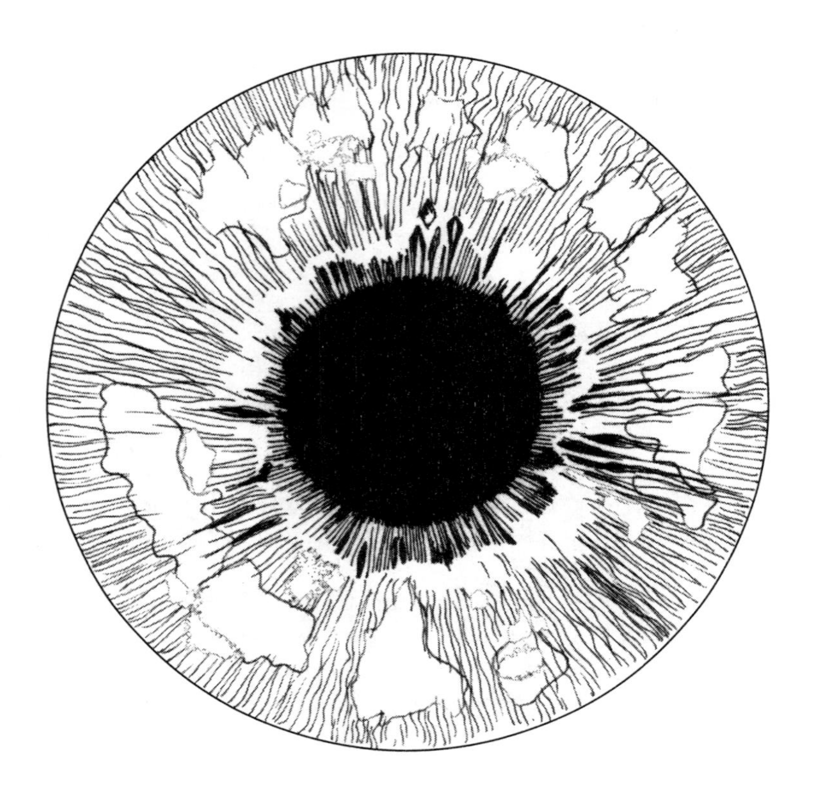

Iris Color	Blue
Fiber Structure	Silk, Linen, Cotton fiber types
Description	Complete or partial circular platelets of lymphatic tophi in the peripheral to central part of the iris up to the collarette
Aging/Disease Pathways	Lymphatic and body tissues
Systems	Lymphatic, urinary, nervous
Other Possible Signs	Large tophi deep in the iris, changes in color from white to gray, yellow or orange over the tophi, gray scurf ring, thick white or colored collarette

Tissue Weakness	Tissues where tophi cover iris areas
Gland Weakness	None unless depicted by other iris signs
Organ Weakness	Kidney and any others depicted by iris signs
Activity	Toxicity, uric acid retention, congestion
Symptoms	Arthritis, gout, kidney problems, rheumatism
Eliminate	Alcohol, meat, salt, dairy foods, processed flour products, inorganic minerals, acid foods
Diet	Fresh raw, steamed or baked vegetables, especially celery and parsley; purification, mono, vegetable juice and alkaline diets are essential; seaweeds are excellent
Lifestyle	Must avoid indulgences and excesses, develop a simple pure lifestyle and devote time to purifying the body, emotions and mind
Herbs	Kidney, Lymphatic, Chronic Purifier, Heavy Metal, Alkaline and Anti–Inflammatory formulae
Treatments	Homeopathic miasmic level treatment; deep tissue massage; Ginger kidney poultices; reflexology

Personality

Because this person is controlled and inhibited by the past and its influence on the present, it is very difficult for them to become themselves. They are shackled by a weight that resists release and transformation. It will be very difficult for this person to be creative or to have the confidence to forge an individual lifestyle. When their system is relieved of the toxic burden they begin to experience their potential for creativity and joy. If they do not free themselves their life will be limited. Either way they will be burdened by the body. The choice to cooperate fully in purification and healing is a better option than suffering increasingly uncomfortable symptoms. If the mind and heart can recognizing that they are a link in the evolutionary chain of life, they will be inspired to do the work of transforming straw into gold.

Challenge

Because this constitution is burdened by inherited toxins these individuasl must be willing to give time and attention to cleansing and freeing themselves from this influence on their body and lives. It is as though there are only two choices: suffer the consequences or be willing to activate elimination and rejuvenation and live a simple, healthy lifestyle.

Glandular Digestive Emotional

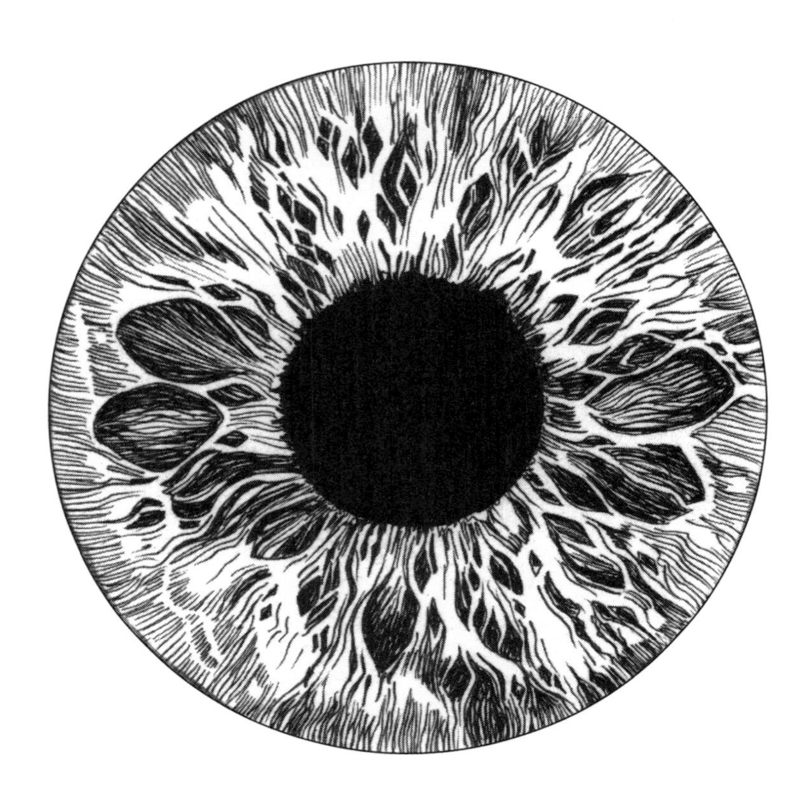

Iris Color	Brown or blue
Fiber Structure	Collarette structure is open, in a regular or irregular pattern. The fibers in the outer iris are structurally stronger
Description	The area outside and beyond the collarette and autonomic nerve wreath, where organs, glands and digestive absorption into blood and lymph takes place, is structurally open in varying patterns, irregularities and shapes
Aging/Disease Pathways	Digestive and nervous systems in the collarette area
Systems	Digestive, endocrine, reproductive, nervous
Other Possible Signs	Central heterachromia, bowel pockets

Tissue Weakness	Bowels, glands, organs, autonomic nervous functions
Gland Weakness	Any gland area where iris fibers open into lacunae
Organ Weakness	Any organ area where iris fibers open into lacunae
Activity	The natural healthy potential of this iris is to release and express; whenever energy is held in, whether it is through constipation on the physical level, repression on the emotional level or introversion on the mental level, it will block movement and release, producing toxicity, sluggish function and inhibition
Symptoms	Constipation, poor digestion, infertility
Eliminate	Rich, heavy foods, eaten late at night, overeating, too many combinations, drinking with meals, insufficient chewing
Diet	Mono diet, simple foods, alkaline cleansing diets, raw fruits and vegetables, high fiber and fresh juices; the main meal of the day should be at noon or no later than 5 p.m.; regular intake of seaweeds and liquid minerals and natural digestive herb teas, papain and chlorophyll will improve digestion
Lifestyle	It is important to exercise after eating; do not sleep on a full stomach; expression and release through creative activities like dancing, art and music are important
Herbs	Bowel Rejuvenator, Nerve Rejuvenator, Hormone, Body Building, Thyroid, Multi–Vitamin Mineral and Calcium formulae
Treatments	Castor oil packs, enemas and abdominal packs

Personality

The structural openings flower into the emotional life, allowing spontaneous feeling. Because they express visually they learn best through voice and sound. When introverted, they are contained inwardly in dreams, fantasies and visions. Fulfillment comes through creative joy.

Challenge

This type needs to learn to take in nourishment, process it, utilize the energy and then release what is not needed. Any inhibition of this flow will cause toxic buildup. It is also essential that this type enjoy and release creativity, color and beauty, as well as to develop concentration and mental organizational structural abilities. Because their energetic pattern is to digest life, the development of discrimination as to what is good for them and what is not, on all levels, is very important. What they cannot digest will cause distress.

Structurally Open

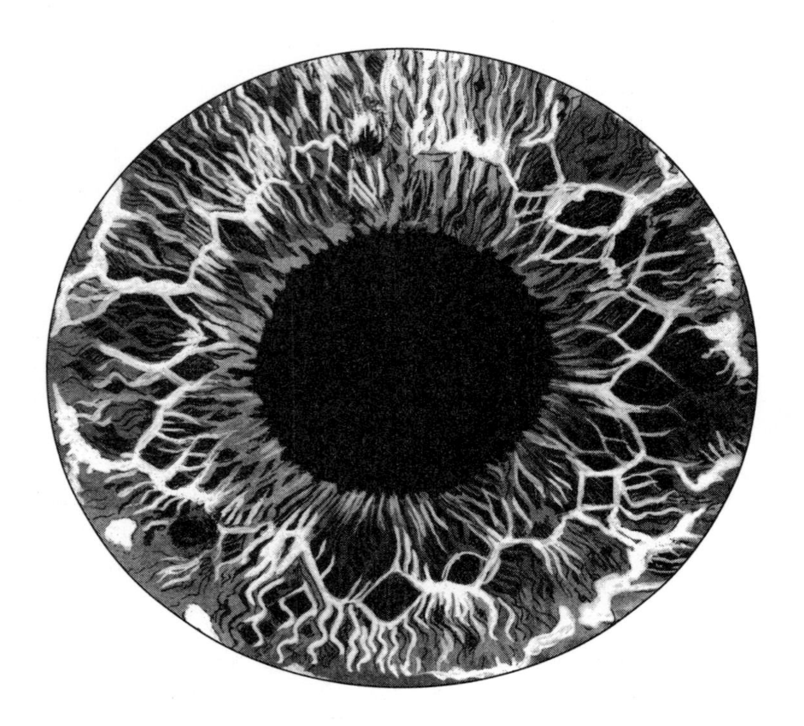

Iris Color	Brown or blue
Fiber Structure	Burlap
Description	The entire iris is covered with flower or leaf lacunae patterns, honeycomb structures, and a loose, hard–to–define collarette
Aging/Disease Pathways	Bone, muscular, glandular and organ structural weakness
Systems	Structural, glandular, digestive
Other Possible Signs	Other signs which may occur over this structure are sensitivity rings, central heterachromia, darkening of lacunae, bowel pockets, crypts, reflexive fibers, dark scurf ring in the skin zone on the iris/sclera margin

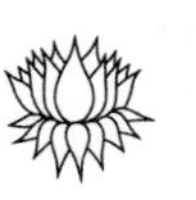

Tissue Weakness	Bowel, muscles, connective tissue
Gland Weakness	Any gland area where a lacunae opens; it is more chronic if there is toxic darkness inside, or more acute if white; the adrenals are often involved
Organ Weakness	Any organ area where a lacunae opens; look for darkening or whitening to indicate toxicity or inflammation
Activity	Bones and muscles are inherently weak and slow to heal or recuperate; they easily become sluggish, fatigued and toxic
Symptoms	Weak bones, joints and muscles cause varicose and spider veins, hemorrhoids, prolapse, hernia, spinal misalignment, poor posture and curvature of the spine and aches and pains
Eliminate	Junk foods, denatured processed foods, stress
Diet	Natural whole food high fiber diet, seaweeds and liquid minerals, fresh vegetables juices
Lifestyle	Moderate living habits, walking, swimming, tai chi, yoga
Herbs	Anemia, Exhaustion, Calcium, Body Building, Adrenal, Bowel Rejuvenator or Vitalizer, Circulation Systemic formulae; Licorice tea, spirulina, algaes, seaweeds
Treatments	Massage, Castor oil packs, chiropractic, osteopathy

Psychology

Strong socially, this type is sensitive, adaptable and communicative. They are at their best in crisis situations or in crowded communities where their compassion, tolerance and understanding make them natural leaders, because their concern is for the welfare of individuals. They do not sacrifice the individual to community goals like the structurally strong leader. Because they live within their own weaknesses and limitations, they understand the weaknesses of others. When negative exhaustion, apathy and fatigue take over, they lose purpose and interest because they don't have the energy to make things happen or to manifest change.

Challenge

This type of person needs to create structure to balance their expressive creativity and instinctual feeling. They need to accept that they will have to care for their bodies, live within its limits and develop a lifestyle that will enable them to enjoy good health.

Circulatory Hardening

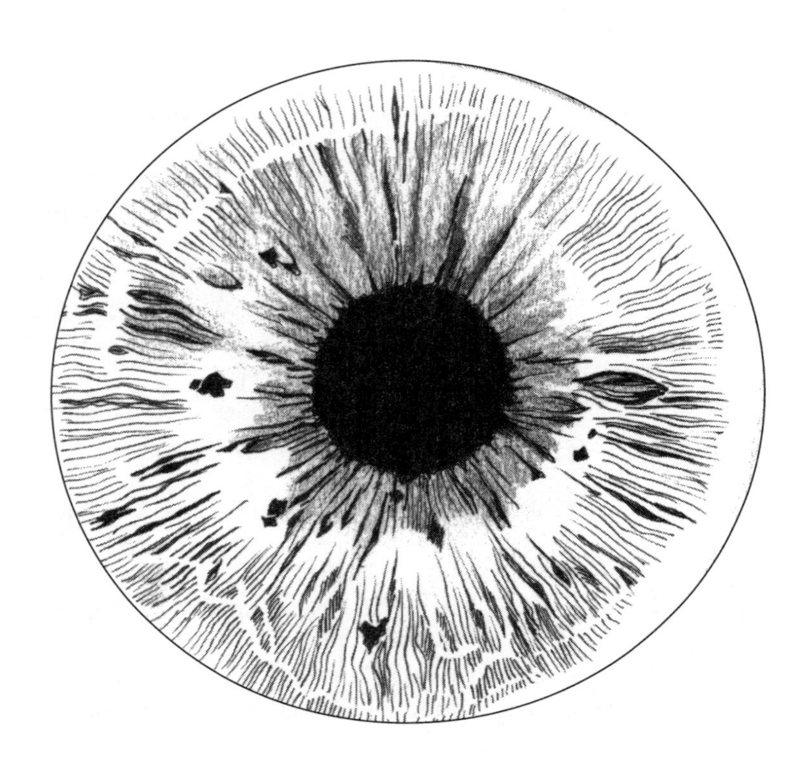

Iris Color	Brown, blue
Fiber Structure	Any fiber structure, or the mixed or velvet brown type
Description	Partial or full white ring of varying widths (translucent to opaque) in the lymphatic, circulatory and skin zones
Aging/Disease Pathways	Inhibition of circulation, calcium imbalances, heart weakness
Systems	Circulatory, lymphatic
Other Possible Signs	Arcus senilis, scurf and sensitivity rings as well as heart, liver, and thyroid indications

Tissue Weakness	Arteries, capillaries, heart
Gland Weakness	Thyroid and parathyroid glands affect calcium imbalances in the blood
Organ Weakness	Heart, liver, spleen, and often kidneys; look for any iris signs
Activity	Blood thickens, reducing peripheral circulation; the liver is overburdened; lymph can't purify fluids; plaguing and hardening of the arteries creates blood pressure imbalances; aging develops through hardening; circulation loss diminishes the flow of life through the body; cholesterol increases; increased calcium buildup in the joints and tissues
Symptoms	Poor circulation, anemia of the extremities, poor concentration and memory, depression, senility, muscle and joint stiffness, high or low blood pressure, arthritis and rheumatism, aches and pains, hearing loss, hypothyroidism, liver dysfunction, cardiovascular degeneration
Eliminate	Salt, alcohol, fat, aspirin, fried foods, inorganic minerals, cholesterol, eggs, meat
Diet	Alkaline, vegetarian, mono diets; raw organic produce, fresh juices, distilled water, seaweeds, garlic, lecithin, vitamin E, liver cleanse drinks
Lifestyle	Exercise, steams and saunas; stay active
Herbs	Systemic treatment: Circulation Systemic and Cerebral, Heart, Lymph, Liver, Blood Purifying and Thyroid formulae; Buckwheat tea
Treatments	Massage; rolfing; tai chi; yoga

Personality

Because the physical level manifests hardening of the arteries and slowing of circulation, lessening vitality and oxygenation, the emotional and mental levels reflect this with inflexibility, resistance, inability to adapt or adjust, domination and unwillingness to change. Because of their fixed nature they can become judgmental, impatient and arrogant, or lost in their own mind, unable to communicate, release or enjoy. They also become depressed when they suffer from an inability to concentrate and have poor memory. Like the pillar of salt they harden body, heart and mind and eventually shut themselves inside. Extreme cases are manic depressive. Others may only experience physical symptoms, which vary greatly from person to person.

Challenge

This type creates a barrier, a white ring representing loss of flexibility together with a lack of interest in the outside world. With a natural tendency to fixed ideas they believe their way is the right way. They need to learn tolerance for different ways of seeing and doing things, compassion and the ability to listen to others. Softening and dissolving are the balances they require. Because this type resists change, their healing and evolution may take longer and require more effort.

Anxiety Gastric

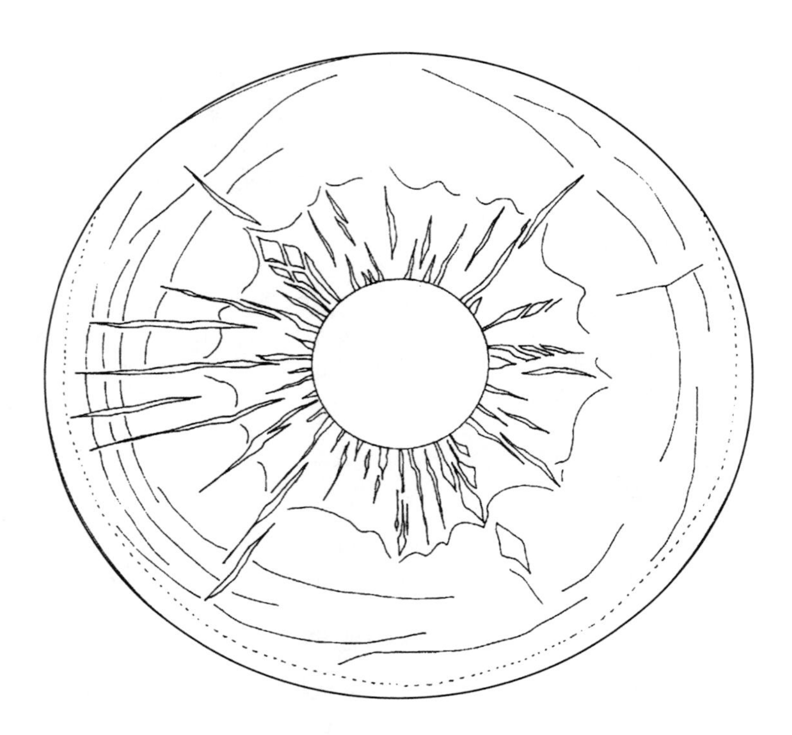

Iris Color	Brown or blue
Fiber Structure	Any fiber structure
Description	Radii soleris radiating out from the center combined with sensitivity rings, in varying patterns, density, and numbers
Aging/Disease Pathways	Digestive and nervous systems affecting each other
Systems	Digestive, nervous, glandular
Other Possible Signs	Toxic radii soleris; radii going through a major organ, gland or brain areas; radii breaking through the collarette affecting the autonomic nervous system; bowel toxicity; acute or toxic sensitivity rings

Tissue Weakness	Wherever radii break through the collarette, or terminate, there is potential weakness in the bowels or autonomic nervous system
Gland Weakness	Any gland the radii run through, such as adrenal, thyroid, pancreas
Organ Weakness	Any organ the radii run through, such as heart, liver, kidney, spleen
Activity	If the bowels are toxic the radii are used to dispense toxins into reflex areas affecting organs, glands, body systems and tissues, causing irritation and hyperactive neuro–muscular activity and psychosomatic ailments blood diseases and calcium imbalances
Symptoms	Angina, anxiety, cardiac stress, colitis, constipation, epilepsy, headaches, hysteria, intestinal spasms, nervous stomach, thyroid deficiency, ulcers
Eliminate	Sugar, fried foods, junk and processed foods, eating on the run, when under stress or during emotional conflicts
Diet	Wholefood vegetarian fresh organic vegetables, fruits, grains, nuts and seeds; fresh vegetable juices; alkaline diet; mono diet
Lifestyle	Must avoid stress; must take care to avoid living in conflict situations; exercise; meditation, tai chi and yoga are recommended
Herbs	Bowel Rejuvenator, Nerve Rejuvenator, Tonic or Vitalizer, Adrenal, Thyroid, Alkaline and the Multi–Vitamin/Mineral Naturally formulae
Treatments	Castor oil pack; Ginger poultice over kidneys; cold abdominal pack; polarity balancing; massage; acupuncture; Bach flower remedies

Personality

This type contains two strong energy movements, outward goal direction through radii soleris, and inward containment through sensitivity rings. In their negative expression this type wallows in unresolved conflict, wastes energy, stops, changes, is unable to make a decision, follow through or resolve problems. Breakdown is the inevitable result of exhausted adrenals and a depleted nervous system. The positive expression is manifested when the person can express and dialogue both aspects of their personality with creative joy, and resolve conflicts by looking at both sides before making the best choice or perhaps doing both. They may avoid choice by going along with whatever stronger, more defined personalities around them want to do.

Challenge

This type needs balance, stillness, inner strength and wisdom. They must learn to dialogue internally, and overcome the tendency to exhaust themselves with situations and conflicts they can't mediate, harmonize or resolve. They must balance their sensitivity so that they are not a victim of this knot of vacillating feelings, or stay where they cannot free themselves from or resolve conflicts.

Mixed Color

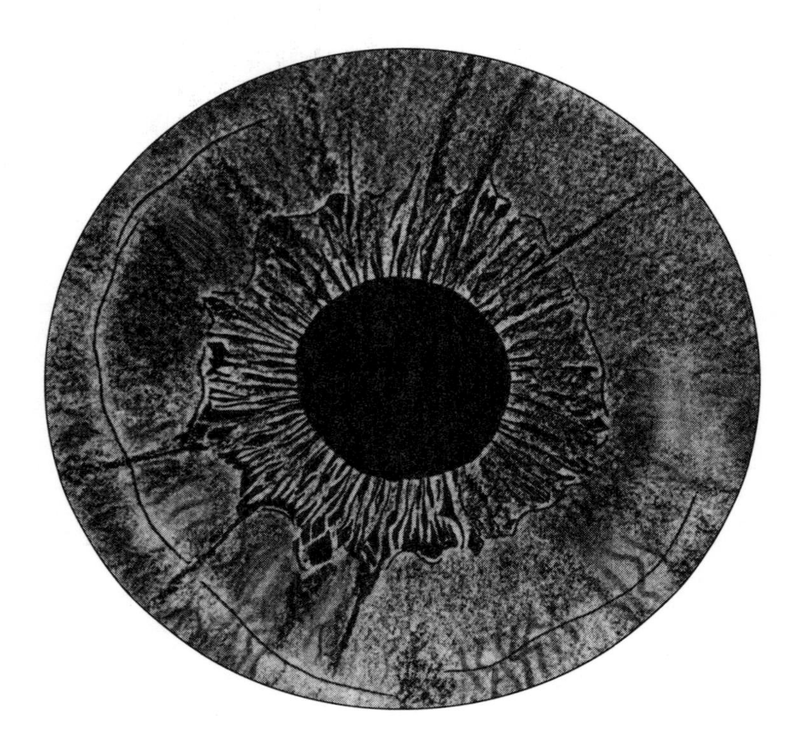

Iris Color	Various shades of brown mixed with blue, yellowish green or greenish blue
Fiber Structure	Mostly light brown velvet without fiber structure with occasional fibers showing in the blue, green, yellow areas, or near the sensitivity rings
Description	Light brown velvet iris with blue or green, yellow or blue revealed in the pelvic areas or near sensitivity rings
Aging/Disease Pathways	Blood, bowels and digestive organs
Systems	Digestive
Other Possible Signs	Central heterachromia, radii soleris, lacunae, sensitivity rings, bowel pockets and organ weakness

Tissue Weakness	Digestive organs, glands and tissues
Gland Weakness	No specific one unless indicated by radii or lacunae
Organ Weakness	No specific one unless indicated by radii or lacunae
Activity	This type blends brown iris aging and disease pathways of digestive and blood toxicity together with blue iris acute reactiveness
Symptoms	Constipation, sluggish digestion, flatulence
Eliminate	Fats, fried foods, rich and complicated combinations
Diet	High fiber, high iron, alkaline diet, low protein and low fat, fresh fruits and vegetables; do not combined fruit with other foods; it is best not to eat fast, late at night or drink excessively with meals; seaweeds are good
Lifestyle	Simple diet, exercise and a moderate work and social life
Herbs	Bowel Rejuvenator, Blood Purifying, Liver/Gall Bladder, Pancreas, Circulation Systemic and the Anemia formulae
Treatments	Castor oil pack

Personality

This type combines a lack of clear boundaries, with the ability to relate to and understand different types of people, making strong purpose and self clarity difficult. They are drawn toward both blue–eyed and brown–eyed natures within themselves and in relationships. Confusion and frustration inhibit their evolution toward their own true nature, which is beyond the opposites. They must learn to integrate, unite and blend. This confusion of self–identification can prevent them from proceeding with study, work and creative goals, so it is essential that this person have the opportunity and support to do this integrative work.

Challenge

This type needs to overcome the confusion of being a mixture of both types and to work on self–identity, purpose and clarity. Ambivalence or apathy is a potential problem which can be overcome by breaking through to a deeper level of instinctual feeling, combined with spirituality, which unifies these two different aspects in their being.

Velvet Brown Type

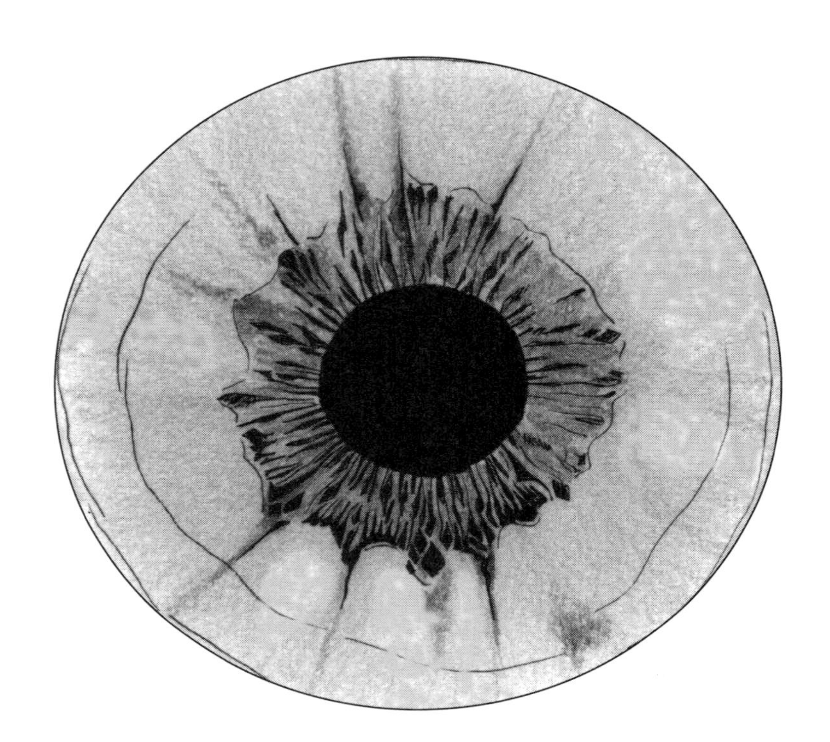

Iris Color	Varying shades of deep velvet brown and brown–black
Fiber Structure	None
Description	Deep brown velvet background on which other iris signs may or may not be displayed
Aging/Disease Pathways	Digestive and blood weaknesses
Systems	Digestive, circulatory
Other Possible Signs	Lacunae, radii soleris, sensitivity rings, different fiber structure inside the collarette, circulatory hardening white ring

Tissue Weakness	Digestive tissues
Gland Weakness	Any gland where lacunae or radii indicate weakness
Organ Weakness	Any organ where lacunae or radii indicate weakness
Activity	Silent pathology accumulates through lack of catalysts (iodine, copper, arsenic, zinc and iron) together with blood making malfunctions, endocrine, organ and digestive problems, and poor elimination
Symptoms	Anemia, blood diseases, constipation, digestive pains and problems, toxicity, spasmodic aches and pains leading to chronic disease
Eliminate	Alcohol, coffee, tea, processed and junk foods, meat, sugar
Diet	Alkaline, vegetarian and purification diets, vegetable juice, chlorophyll, hydrochloric acid, seaweeds, liquid minerals, vitimin B12
Lifestyle	Must have an active natural lifestyle that includes regular exercise, purification and healthy elimination
Herbs	Bowel Rejuvenator, Liver/Gall Bladder, Alkaline, Anemia, Hormone, Calcium and Blood Purifier formulae; drink Red Clover, Red Raspberry and Yellow Dock herbal infusions
Treatments	Castor oil packs, enemas and colonics as required; massage; reflexology

Personality

Healthy individuals of this type are community minded family people who do their duty and contribute to their best ability. When negative, this type becomes obsessive, desires rule them and emotions set their inner and outer worlds off balance. Their mind revolves around unresolved confusion and negative repetitions.

Challenge

Because this type progresses toward disease silently, without acute reactions or aches and pains, it is essential to develop a healthy lifestyle to prevent the development of chronic disease. They need to stay tuned into their body and make sure that it functions well and eliminates completely. Prevention of physical, emotional and mental problems is essential for a moderate daily life. Toxins must not be allowed to accumulate on any level. Emotional suppression is a major problem in the dark–eyed cultures, in extended families in India, China, Africa, and other third world countries. Rather than internalizing and containing their life experience, they need to learn to communicate, release and express. They must keep their bodies functioning and eliminating on a daily basis and strive to take care of their own needs, as well as taking care of others and surrendering to family expectations, duties and commitments.

IRIDOLOGY CHART

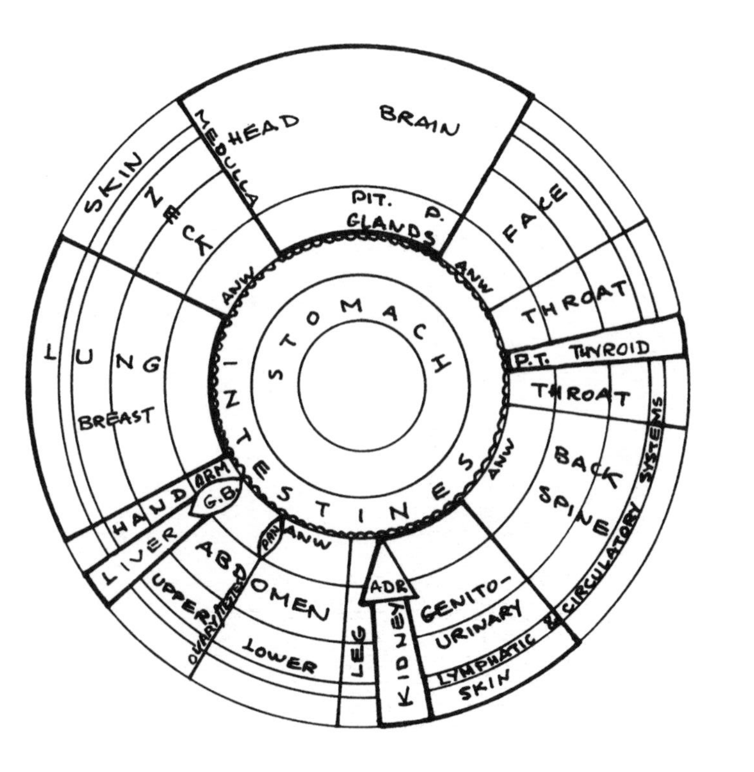

Right Iris

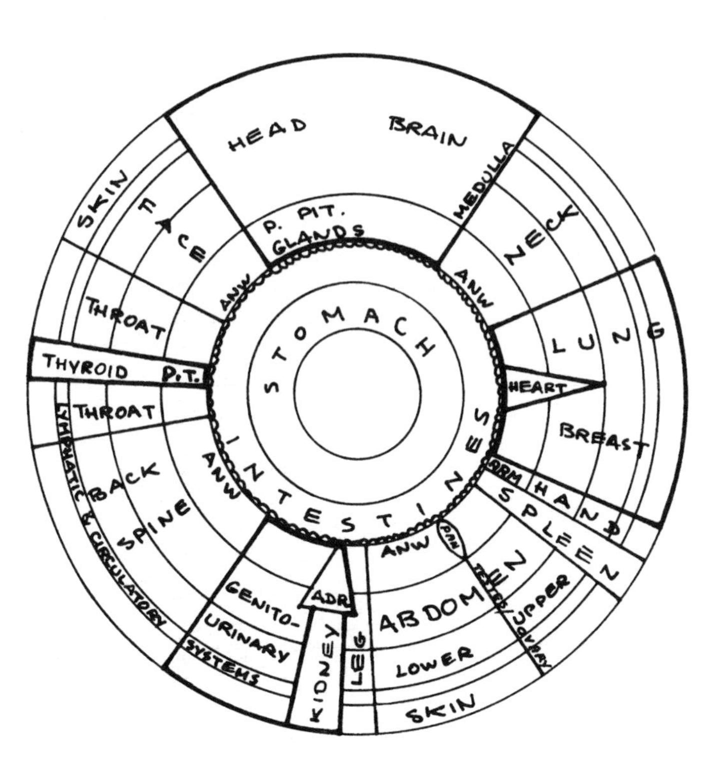

Left Iris

8

Healing Grace

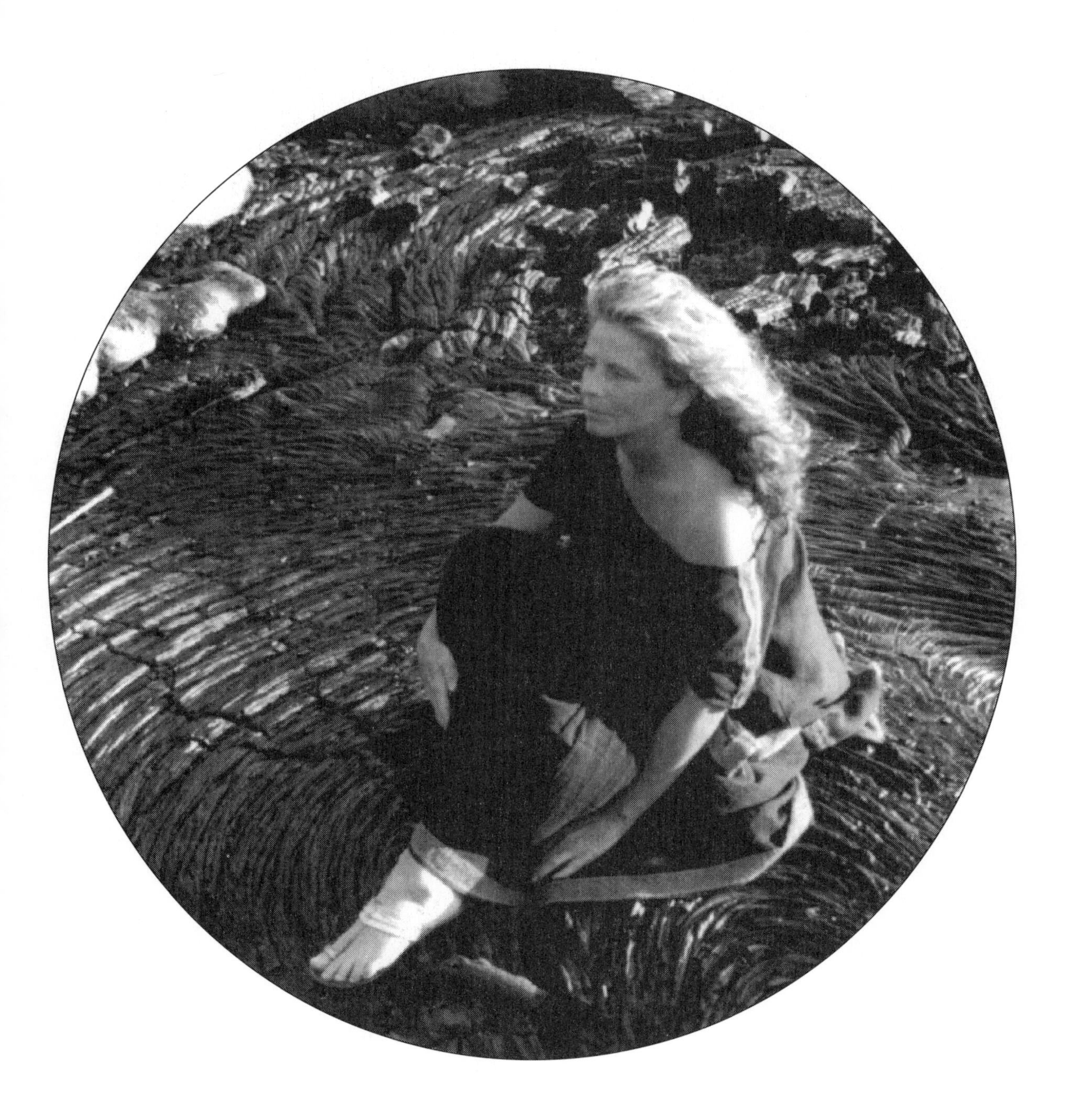

Healing Grace

Now that the time has come to share my story of the unfolding of my life as a spiritual being on this mother planet Earth, I look back and realize that there was only love. During my difficult time, my suffering and my pain, I did not experience it as love. I felt unloved, isolated, separate and alone, unnourished by both human and divine companionship. I did not realize then how constant and present was the loving grace and support that I received as I was shaped and formed throughout my life destiny, so that the light of my consciousness would awaken and shine both within my being and in my daily life. I relate this story in the hope that others may find relief from their suffering by recognizing the divine plan at work in their lives. I also wish to share through my books, workshops and practice the unique processes my heart, mind and spirit created to help me resolve problems as I sought each new level of emergence, so that others may benefit from their healing grace.

Some of the most important events in my life helped create the archetypal roles I have lived during the past twenty–five years, first as the wounded woman, then the self healer, the medicine woman and now the woman of wisdom. I honor, respect and love the pain and sorrow that enabled me to become aware of the wisdom within my being, so that I could serve others, and continue to grow and evolve. I give thanks for the light of consciousness that reaches deeply into every cell of my being, so that when my time comes to leave this body and this planet, I will offer back only light and love to my creator, and release the elements of my being to dance freely as they return to their source.

My life began during springtime blossoming in May 1942 in a humble home, with a mother and father who came together to create a home and a family, but who never really knew each other, never really talked to each other and never really loved each other. I was raised in their home, absorbing their resentments, their grudges, their loneliness and their longing. Like a flower I came into their life, finding nourishment in nature or in books or within myself, for it was not found in my family, which was without peace, contentment, touch, truth or affection. I escaped into dreams and books and grew as a wildflower, in raw, rough soil that proved, despite its seeming barrenness, fertile ground for a profoundly meaningful life.

Through childhood and teenage years I experienced emptiness and loneliness as well as a longing for love in a life that seemed devoid of nourishment, companionship and guidance. My life destiny provided the opportunity to create my illnesses and then to heal them through a series of mystical coincidences and divine synchronicities which were supported by my use of herbs and nature cure. Both the suffering and the gift of healing opened the potential of my life work as a medicine woman. Through wisdom and experience, my life expanded into a wider horizon of profound purpose, satisfaction, and relationship. I created an authentic path and began the spiritual journey to my heart's goal of true and lasting divine nourishment. Because of the grace of my life journey, the transformation of difficulties into purpose gives me great joy.

I know now that true nourishment comes only from within. All attempts to seek nourishment and love from others and from material things give only temporary satisfaction, purpose or excitement. I was empty and hungry both inwardly and outwardly as a child and young woman. Now, because I no longer look, long for or expect nourishment to come from outside myself, I can give love, service and nourishment without thought of return and find peace and contentment in this life as I live in gratitude for the gifts, love and abundance that surround me.

If nourishment does come from another person or a circumstance outside myself I can receive, accept, and enjoy it, but also let it go. If we are able to receive what is being given because we are not blinded by longing for something else, we can live daily life in gratitude, contentment and simplicity. This is the greatest gift. We can be happy and at home anywhere. The ability to sense, know, accept and use nourishment is the key to the spiritual life which combines instinct, ancient wisdom and simplicity.

I share my story as a gift to those who seek healing evolution and long to discover and live the mystery of their highest purpose as it unfolds. I give thanks to my self–healing experience and the years I have served as a medicine woman. These years taught me, on many levels, the importance of nourishment and our ability to open to it, receive it, digest it and make it part of our lives. Our journey as a human being begins and ends with nourishment. Our longing for nourishment, where we seek it and what we do with it, is the story of our lives. Here is my story.

Wildflower

One sunny summer afternoon when I was about five years old I was sitting on the front steps of our house on the hill overlooking the seaside town of White Rock, British Columbia. The air was fragrant and warm. Bees were buzzing. I remember wondering why all the grownups wanted to shut themselves away in a dim room, smoking and playing cards, away from all this light. Radiance beamed from the abundance of full summer and the glory of green and other brilliant colors captured my heart in a dream of beauty. Quite absentmindedly I reached out and picked a leaf. As I brought it near me I inhaled the fragrance of lemon. Lemon? I was struck with amazement and surprise. How could a plant smell like a lemon? I jumped up, unable to contain my delight and rushed inside.

"Mommy. Daddy. I found a lemon plant. Look. Smell. Lemon. It's lemon." I had interrupted their card game. Everyone turned to look at me. I became self–conscious and shy and backed away.

"It's just an herb, dear," my father said kindly. "Now, run and play." They went back to their game and I returned to the dazzling, sunlit garden. I sat on the steps in deep thought, pondering the plant, holding it, looking at it, smelling it, chewing it. A plant that was a lemon. What a mystery.

When the guests left later, one elderly lady sat down beside me and told me that herbs were gifts from God and that many of them had special virtues that helped and healed people. She

explained that this plant, Lemon Verbena, made a pleasant tea that people liked to take not only for its lovely fragrance and taste, but because it was soothing and helped digestion.

"Could I drink it? Could I? Would it be good for me?" I questioned passionately. The idea that this lemon plant had a purpose made me even more excited.

"Yes, dear. Ask your mother to make you a drink tonight."

"I will. I will. Oh, thank you, thank you," I called to her as she waved goodbye and walked down the flowering path towards the garden gate.

I did have my lemon drink that night, savoring the taste as well as the awakening of the mystery of nature and plants. A new world opened to me that day. Nature became a frontier of wonders and miracles for my explorations of curiosity. From that day I received a conscious love and trust of nature and her healing plants that have remained with me all my life. This attitude of awe and respect for creation, for healing plants and their abilities to help humankind, formed the basis of my life's work as an herbalist.

As my childhood years sped by, I played happily on the beach, in the sea, the forest and in the meadows. I was a child of nature, up early in the summer to run and play until the sunset forced me to return home to bath and bed. My favorite game was playing 'Indians' with my brother and sisters. We created dwellings out of sticks and twigs, made clay pots which we used for pretend meals of freshly picked plants and herbs. My brother and I dug happily through mounds of clam shells the native Indians had left on Crescent Beach in British Columbia, finding tools, arrowheads, mortars and pestles which we used in our games. In the evenings I was an avid reader of novels about primitive peoples, Indians and cultures from far away. I spent many hours pouring over National Geographic magazines, imagining what it would be like to live close to nature, and envying the color, costumes, community and communion with the natural world.

During my teenage years my family moved to Vancouver, leaving behind the country life. I went to high school and became caught up in studies and student life. Sociability and dating were difficult and awkward for me because of my shyness and self–consciousness. I was always more comfortable alone, reading, bicycling, skating, going on my own to movies, studying and taking dance classes. These activities made me happy and I soon became a loner. I never found a friend who could share my world.

This lack of social grace and personal power led me into an early marriage because I did not know how to say 'no' to a man who wanted me. I had no skills with which to guide my own life. My gentle nature which longed to give and receive love, to serve and to please was helpless before the dominant creative energy of my husband. I became lost in his life and surrendered all that I loved: solitude, books, dance, movies, nature, spirituality and study. Because he did not want me to do anything that I loved, I forgot who and what I was or even what I loved to do.

It was only when I became pregnant that my interest in natural ways resurfaced and I found myself announcing to husband, family and friends that I was going to have a happy, natural birth like the Indians. They humored me, but I know that they secretly thought that when faced with the realities of giving birth I would scream for anaesthesia and talk about how painful it was for the rest of my life. From within my being I believed that giving birth was natural and beautiful

and I was determined that it would be that way for me. During the pregnancy I blossomed with a sense of inner truth and knowing. Strength rose up in me that gave me the courage and determination to experience giving birth according to my vision.

I searched and finally found a doctor (this was 1963 and natural childbirth was virtually unknown in Vancouver at that time) who had visited Russia on a fellowship where he had observed natural childbirth. At least he knew it was possible. I had to settle for that. I ordered a translation of a French book on natural childbirth, and while it wasn't exactly inspiring, it did mention breathing techniques and the realities of birth. I never met one woman who gave me encouragement or provided me with information to help or guide me. I only heard complaints. I had to practice on my own. During this time, however, my sense of joy and love was great. I had never been happier. I was bringing my child into the world and this was the most beautiful thing that had ever happened to me. I spent hours each day communing with my child within, talking, singing, imagining, and welcoming him into my life. I felt his presence within me and, difficult as my life was with my husband, no outward troubles lessened my excitement and joy.

As destiny would have it, there were complications. The water broke early, almost a month premature. I was admitted into the hospital but as full labor didn't start until a week later, I was in a state of constant expectation and excitement. Once labor started the birth moved quickly. I breathed through the waves of cramps and was able to relax and enjoy the opening of the pelvis. My whole world became those surging waves, opening, opening. I found that the breathing, combined with a particular chanting sound took any pain away. The head crowned. It didn't hurt. I only felt hot. I panted to let the tissues take their time to stretch the vaginal opening and then my son came into this world, and I was laughing and crying as the birth attendants handed him to me. Nothing mattered except this love and this joy, and I felt victorious because the birth had been beautiful and natural.

This experience of motherhood, the birthing, nursing, loving and caring for my infant son, gave me a sense of my own power, of what I felt was truth and the way I felt life should be. I began to have a sense of my own inner world. As the years passed by, I had two more awe–inspiring births and brought two more beautiful children into a modern world that resisted natural ways. In my marriage I struggled against a husband who could not open to the love and joy of family life. My inner sense of strength and purpose grew stronger, and my search for love and the natural way became my goal in life. If one area of my life resisted my need to give and receive love, like Mercury, my birth sign, I moved in another direction, always towards love.

We had moved to California in December 1963, after the birth of Galon, my first child, and over the next two years my husband and I opened art galleries in Carmel, on La Cienega in Los Angeles, and in Scottsdale, Arizona. I proved capable of managing the galleries, hanging shows, photographing art, writing brochures and selling. This natural talent flowered as the challenges presented themselves. I also helped with the sculptures, learning how to weld. Creativity blossomed during this period. I had found another ground of confidence. I began to design and make my own clothes and jewelry, fulfilling a need for clothes that allowed me to feel comfortable, expressed how I felt, and let me move freely.

FLOWER CHILD

During the sixties our studio in Santa Monica became a psychedelic playground for the flower children of L.A. We created a strangely beautiful environment with silver mirrored floors and curving panels of silver, gold and colored reflecting mylar on which my husband's sculptures were placed. Ultra–violet lights, strobes, slides and filtered colored lights created an ambience of psychedelic outer space. In our studio the real world was left behind. Parties, TV producers, art dealers, clients, rock groups, the brotherhood of man and the flower children came and went. Love and peace flowed and LSD opened up visions of the unity of all life and the sanctity of nature. Then the atmosphere of this magic time changed. The excitement of the love, the costumes, the fantasy head trips, communes, free food kitchens, pied piper rock band messages, psychedelic light and sound shows and all the visionary stimulation of flower power lost its innocence as indulgence in free love and drugs involved police and the FBI, who brought a sinister fear and darkness to the counter–revolution. Paranoia began to overshadow love.

Always seeking love, I escaped to a commune in the Valley and spent delight–filled weeks being one of the 'Beautiful People' living out the song 'All you need is Love.' I had been drawn to a group of robed men and women at the Renaissance Faire. An aura of love and beauty radiated from them, so I sat with them, drinking it in. When the next Faire was cancelled, I was heartbroken. How would I find them again? After nearly six weeks I finally saw them at the Griffith Park Love In. They had been looking for me as well. The attraction was magnetic. I drove home with them to the Valley, singing along to the car radio, playing Jim Morrison's latest hit song, 'Light my Fire, 'as I entered a new world of communal love, friendship and fun.

Kent, Mary, and their flower children brothers and sisters invited my children and me into their life. Every day we played, created art, danced, and swam at Malibu beach or in the pool at the waterfall. My new friends surrounded me with love. I had never been so happy, nor enjoyed life so much. The intense productive success–oriented work life and the creative chaos of my husband's art studio and boutique vanished. I didn't want to return home, but eventually my husband persuaded me. I wept as I left behind what I had experienced as my first true family of love.

The return to my old lifestyle was impossible. I had changed. Problems in my marriage that had been suppressed for years surfaced. Now, instead of going along with everything submissively, I had a new vision and wanted a different and better life. I wanted love and happiness, not just work. I wanted true friends who cared for me, not customers. My husband did not want to change, and I could not return to my old life. The very core of my being resisted going backward, but I did not know what to do.

As if in answer to my longing, I received an invitation to visit a community in Hawaii. After months of running my boutique, the Psychedelic Conspiracy on Sunset Strip, where I created costumes for Love Ins, the Renaissance Faire and rock bands, I felt totally burnt out because the 'love generation' had become the 'sex and drug generation.' I no longer wanted to be part of what was happening. I left husband, store and studio and escaped to Hawaii in the summer of 1967 to merge with the soft, fragrant, succulent Mother earth and sea and flow into the fantasy of paradise. I didn't want any more metal, plastic, or Sunset Strip hype. I wanted Mother Nature to take me in her arms and hold me, comfort me and heal me. I wanted and needed nourishment for myself on every level.

With an open, seeking consciousness I awakened to nature and recognized for the first time the dance of the elements of earth, water, fire, air and ether. This dance of nature helped me to understand cycles, seasons and transformation: birth and death, death and birth, in continuum. Life was energy. I recognized instinctively that nature was wisdom, ready to reach out and speak and teach if we would only look and listen.

I lived on a farm in Haiku, which was one day destined to become a Buddhist Zendo. Here I lived out my fantasy of paradise. My oldest daughter, Casel, born in 1966, was with me, a golden cherub of one and a half years. We dressed in flowing fabrics, long dresses, shawls and capes, and put flowers in our hair. Each day we walked to the waterfall to play and swim together in the flower–filled water of the guava–scented grotto. We sat together in the quiet majesty of the eucalyptus grove, absorbing the healing peace while the fragrance purified the air as it played around us. Whenever we met native Hawaiians they begged to adopt Casel. She was pure, sweet and unbelievably beautiful, an angel flower child.

I collected eucalyptus buds, strung them into necklaces and sewed them on my clothes. I began to sense that plants, trees and flowers became outward manifestations of a subtle spiritual radiance, vibratory essences that reached outward and became leaves, seeds, buds and flowers. I saw the light and the spirit of the Creator around every living thing and realized that we are all a part of the radiant flow of light, love and life. I felt the presence of the ancient Hawaiians shining down upon us, and nature became so alive and abundant to me that man–made metal and concrete appeared dead and cold in contrast.

Because of these illuminations I yearned to learn nature's secrets. The more I loved nature, the more it spoke to me and guided me. Each hill was a temple, each cloud a message from the divine. I experienced how the primitives and Indians honored, feared and respected nature. My mind opened to a new dimension of perceiving life, directly through my senses, faculties and intuition. My whole being absorbed wisdom from nature on a deep inner primal level, beyond the intellect. I wandered through the Hawaiian countryside, guided by signs in the landscape and my intuition and discovered old temples, rare plants and sacred places. I carried my third child, Chalice, within me during this time of awakening my goddess within.

One special day a friend, a golden yoga teacher I had met when staying with Kent and Mary, arrived from California to bring me the sacrament from the White Brotherhood near Laguna. We climbed a sacred hill that overlooked a turquoise bay dancing with white waves, to an orchard bordered with stately palms. He watched over me while I went into the most

exquisite state of being, spontaneously assuming a pose, the right hand stretched upward facing outward in giving, and the left hand facing outward in the gesture of receiving. So exquisite and perfect was this pose, that I never moved from this position all day. I found out later that it was the pose of Kwan Yin, the goddess of compassion.

During this spiritually uplifted state, my gaze opened to the light–filled heaven–sky, and the fresh movement of cloud patterns gave messages of love that danced through the flowering trees and whispered amongst the grasses. Each moment was absolute perfection. The wind from the sea expressed the truth of God's love. Clouds swirled into divine visions that blessed me with grace. The earth clinging to my bare feet felt distant, dark, moist and coarse. As sunset approached I heard my friend call my name. I turned toward his voice and looked upward into a tree of glowing blossoms where he was watching over me. Slowly, reluctantly we departed, stopping to bathe in a waterfall pool where I lay suspended like a bubble on the surface, inhaling the fragrance of guava and the sunset skies. We baked dry on hot rocks, absorbing the strength of stone energy before we climbed the path homeward through the fragrant violet–starred dusk settling mysteriously over the lush leafy green tropical landscape.

When I entered the farmhouse I caught a glimpse of myself in a mirror. My face was burnt nearly black from standing in the face of the sun all day. My friend and I were so full of divine love and grace we couldn't eat, so we sat in my room in meditation, feeling a pull that took us inward toward our God Self. With soulfulness I read out loud from Kahlil Gibran and felt the power and the truth of the words as I held the book with deep respect. How blessed I felt to be able to experience such a state of consciousness. That night I slept on a cloud of happiness and fulfillment and the joy lasted for days. I will never forget the potential of the divine feminine and the blessing of this goddess, Kwan Yin.

Toward the end of September, I took a spiritual pilgrimage up Haleakala, the 'House of the Sun,' Maui's largest volcano that rises up from the sea and dominates the island. The commune members agreed to take care of Casel, while Bro, Lion and Steve joined me on our volcano vision quest. We hitchhiked across the island to the base of the Haleakala to begin our ascent. All day we walked slowly through the rising changes of vegetation, the land becoming more and more barren, and the air cooler and cooler, until it appeared that we were no longer in tropical Hawaii. When we paused and looked down, we saw the brilliant green–blue sea edged by frothy white waves enclosing the shore and verdant jungles on the Hana rainforest side. A chill engulfed us as we walked into misty clouds amidst sparse pine trees, and I put on my cloak covered with eucalyptus beads and shells. Even the growing discomfort could not diminish the excitement, because we were on our way to Haleakala, House of the Sun, the ancient Hawaiian volcano lunar landscape.

Dusk came and we were still far from the summit. We clothed ourselves in layers of sweaters and jeans, but the air was bitterly cold now that the sun had vanished. Just as we realized that we were in a dilemma, as if by providence, a truck came up the hill and stopped. It was the forest ranger. After muttering, "Crazy kids," he offered us a ride to the top and we leapt with gratitude into the back of his truck for a ride to the summit of Haleakala.

We passed through the swirling mists to the top of the volcano where the sky was brilliant, relentlessly clear, and sparkling with diamond stars, but the air was so sharp and cold it made our lungs ache. We ran for the stone shelter but found little relief. All night we paced, stamping our feet and rubbing each others' backs, arms and legs. Sleep was impossible, so unbearable was the cold. The longer the separation from the sun and warmth, the greater our longing became for the sun. The early hours of the morning seemed beyond endurance. We could hardly move by then, our bodies were so stiff with the cold. We tried to weep, but our tears froze. Every second seemed stretched by physical agony, and we wondered if the sun would ever rise.

Suddenly we saw a glimmer of light. Excitement filled our hearts as we searched with our eyes and questioned each other, "Is that light? Look, look, it is light!" Yes, the sun had returned to us. We screamed and jumped and hugged each other, crazy with joy for each ray of the returning warmth as it thawed our stiff limbs and brought feeling back to our bodies. The full sunrise gloried in a clear blue sky, but while the sun rose the full moon still hung in the sky. In one direction we faced the glowing sun and in the other the luminous moon. It was as if the long cold night of longing had prepared me for this illumination, one in which I not only absorbed the power and magnificence of the universe, but also one in which I felt the union of the sun and the moon within my being.

The experience of this mystery of the universe created a profoundly deep effect upon me and I wandered off to search out a quiet space. I saw a pile of rocks and headed for them, wanting only to lie down in the full heat of the sun. When I arrived at the rocks I realized they were the remnants of an ancient building and that I had come to yet another sacred place. I lay down and opened to the sun, welcoming it and allowing it to penetrate my being, easing the stiffness and exhaustion as I drifted into a trance that lifted me into a heaven of joyous laughing Hawaiians amidst a flower–filled land of happiness, beauty and abundance. They welcomed me with their shining faces and we played as children in paradise together.

Eventually I heard voices calling me and I slowly emerged from my visions. I felt sad that I had to return to the present. Lion came over the hill and called out. "There you are. We've been looking for you. We have a ride down the hill."

I got up and quietly walked back to the stone house where tourists and cars now filled the space of our holy pilgrimage night. Soon we were in a car heading for Lahaina. Like a treasure, I carried the feminine mystery of paradise and the balance of sun and moon within me, and did not want to speak or open my eyes. When we reached Lahaina, I asked them to drop me off by the banyan tree. I lay on a bench beneath its benevolent protection and then walked over to a park by the shore where I could lean against a palm tree and gaze outward toward the ocean. I wanted to remain as long as possible in this beautiful state of consciousness.

As I sat in the grass, long hair wild and curling in the wind, flowering dress and cloak draped about me, I noticed a sailboat arriving and watched curiously as the two sailors screamed and yelled with happiness. They pulled up at the dock and raced over to me, kneeling down in front of me, and laughing as they bowed down their heads at my feet.

"Oh, Queen of Hawaii, we greet you from far off lands," they shouted and then they laughed and rolled around on the ground. A crowd gathere. So lively and bizarre was their

behavior. Then they picked flowers and threw them all over me. When Lion and Bro returned, we discovered the young men had sailed from California and this was the first land they had seen for weeks. Someone in the crowd said that this park was the site of the royal family of Maui and that this was where ancient Hawaiian queens used to welcome visitors. It seemed almost as if we were reliving some past life so that the pure essence of the Hawaii Aloha spirit could flower in the present day. I played the part of the Hawaiian queen, greeting the young men, inquiring after their journey and offering them refreshments. The magic of this encounter remains a treasured memory for me, coming as it did after the vision on Haleakala. I felt as though an ancient island goddess had awakened within me.

The autumn season passed, winter storms arrived, the cycles moved and I returned to L.A. with a deeper and richer interior life that supported me through the final stages of pregnancy. I could not say why I had to return. I just woke up one morning in Haiku, Maui, and knew it was time to leave and I followed this instinct even though it was incredibly difficult to leave Hawaii.

My time in Hawaii took me into my essence, opened visions of beauty, grace, healing and spirituality, but it also made me aware of how isolated and unbalanced I was within my being. I reflected on my years of marriage, my divorce, and my struggles to establish my own life, and I realized for the first time that I had deep emotional problems. I had never talked about myself or shared my pain, but always kept everything locked up inside. While my spiritual self longed to reach up and flow into union with divine love, my earthly heart and mind seemed a labyrinth of pain and unconsciousness. I realized also that I needed help. What kind of help I did not know, but I knew instinctively I could not carry the burden alone any longer. It was killing me.

Lotus Flower, Lotus Seed

Because of this realization I knew I could not return to my husband, the boutique or the art studio, so I accepted an invitation to stay with the rock star, Jim Morrison and his girlfriend Pam, for a few weeks, and then moved in with Judith Brewer, the paper clothes fashion designer who had carried my jewelry designs in her Beverly Hills store. She drew me into her Buddhist group, and the Shakamuni Buddha teachings of the Nichirin Shoshu organization from Japan, who chanted Nam Myoho Renge Kyo and the Lotus sutra. I loved the chanting and the rituals, and I flowed without resistance into the chanting and meetings, totally receptive and feminine, longing only to develop spirituality and to face the difficult realities of my life.

Judith and I chanted through my labor and I experienced a most beautiful and ecstatic birthgiving of my third child, my daughter, Chalice. Despite my joy, life as a single parent with three children created new challenges. Hard as the daily realities were, I devoted myself for four years to the intense daily practice of Buddhism and my duties as a group leader. I took two pilgrimages to the mother temple in Japan where I journeyed inwardly into states of spiritual

communion as the vibrations of the chanting transformed my being. My inner life always seemed so rich, I wondered if I would ever be able to experience the same love and joy in my outward life.

We were told by the Buddhist leaders that chanting would pay off our bad karma and that working for *kosen rufu*, or world peace, would help us purify our lives. Now that I realized that I had bad karmas, the knowledge awoke a part of me that had been unconscious. For the first time I felt a dark and heavy shame when I contemplated what I had endured during my marriage. When I met couples who lived normal lives and who enjoyed family life, I felt keenly the loss of this love, support and cooperation. Painful as this truth was, I attempted to establish a 'normal life' for myself and my children.

I channeled my spirituality into chanting and working to create a home and a job that would support me and my two daughters. My ex-husband took my son and dropped out in the Caribbean in a houseboat, not to return to my life for several years. The magic and the visions got left behind as did the hippies, flower children, being an artist and a designer, and all my old friends and contacts. They were all sacrificed to this so–called 'normal' daily life. Sincere and ready as I was to work off my bad karmas, other challenges emerged. I found I could not refuse aggressive and domineering Nichirin Shoshu leaders who wanted me to go out night after night to do *shakubuku* (find new converts) and lead meetings. I allowed myself to be forced to leave my daughters in the care of babysitters while I worked for Nichirin Shoshu every evening after I got home from my secretarial job. The benefits of the chanting were apparent, but it was a difficult life that imprisoned me, and I longed to escape the unreasonable domination of the leaders. Spirituality and control were intertwined, and as much as I loved the spirituality, the control was damaging to my life. However, I was not yet strong enough to leave.

During this time my passion for chanting created small and large miracles in my life. We were told that we could chant for anything we desired, and that by chanting we would pay off the karma connected with receiving whatever it was we needed or wanted. For some time I chanted only for enlightenment, thinking that to chant for practical things would be a sacrilege to spirituality. The struggle of raising children without a car, without money, or my own home, however, became so difficult that one day I sat down and chanted for a car. After an hour or so, the phone rang and it was my ex–husband asking if I needed a car. Within another hour the car was outside the door. Next I chanted for a home and someone offered me a job that included an apartment. If I became ill I chanted the illness away. I chanted to go on pilgrimage to Japan and childcare and money appeared to make the trip possible. I chanted to heal a severe motorcycle burn that had blistered, and two hours later there wasn't a mark on my leg. It was wonderful and it was scary. But never during four years of chanting for a good, kind, and loving husband did one appear in my life. That was one karmic destiny that chanting was not able to change.

When the leaders' domination of my life became unbearable, I beat their system by vowing to chant six hours a day until I was released. At the three month mark, full of incredible strength, positivity and clarity, I walked into a meeting that was both a celebration of my birthday and a special event that marked my next promotion in leadership, looked at everyone, walked out and never went back. It was such a shock to the group that no one called me or came

to see me. Even though I lived in Santa Monica for years afterwards I never met any of the group again. The door closed on that chapter of my life and a new one opened. I rejoiced in my newfound privacy and freedom, and a life that belonged to me once more.

Seeking Flower

As daily life and spirituality came closer and reflected each other, my mind began to seek knowledge. To fulfill this seeking, I returned to college in 1971 to study anthropology, psychology and philosophy. Passionately in love with knowledge, I studied far into the night while horizons and vistas opened before my seeking mind. During this time I also continued my interest in natural living and experimented with herbs bought from the Back to Eden health food store that had opened in Venice, California. I joined a yoga class and tried my first juice fast, took Golden Seal and Cayenne herbs to purify my body and began to run on the beach. Guarana, a brain stimulant herb, helped me through my studies, and my 4.0 average brought me scholarships and grants.

Through the day care center I was invited to a luncheon where the keynote speaker was Leo Buscaglia. His talk on love and his warm enthusiasm struck a deep chord within me and when I went up to thank him, he invited me to attend his Love Class at the University of California. After four years in Nichirin Shoshu, I had become unused to touch, warmth, love, or communication. It was difficult to go to the class and open up amongst people I did not know. I struggled against fear, shyness, inhibitions and inexperience, particularly when we were asked to share our thoughts and feelings. Slowly I began to open up. Dr. Buscaglia's group made a lasting impression on my consciousness and gave me a vision of family and community love that was based on truthful communication and the honoring of each person's feelings. As wonderful as this experience was, it only made me more aware of the lack of intimacy and support in my life, other than what I received from my children.

During this time I was elected President of the Santa Monica Childcare Mother's Association. Because I was studying political science at college I took my duties seriously and began to research the laws to help the women discover what our group purpose was. When I uncovered abuses and deprivation of mother's rights and brought them before the administrators, I faced firsthand the demons of power. The director told me straight to my face that although we had lawful rights they weren't going to let us use them as it would interfere with their way of doing things. It was either war or capitulation. I chose not to use my energy to fight because I realized that laws and politics were merely an illusion and another tangent away from my spiritual path. I also realized that if I chose to fight I would become part of their power struggles. This I did not want to do. Because I depended on child care and wanted to preserve my respect for the teachers and administrators who have helped me and my children so much, as well as remain true to myself, I resigned as president. The veils of illusion had lifted and I began to see

the hidden motives and realities behind the smiling faces. I also realized that politics was not my path, because even when you are fighting for a worthy cause, you become entangled in a worldly mesh of power and struggle with people who play by their own rules.

After a year and a half of intense scholarship level studies, my body broke down as unresolved emotional traumas associated with the separation and divorce from my children's father surfaced in disease. When my marriage ended and I chose my own life, I did not know how to clear the pain of my separation, grief or loss. Alone, without aid from husband or family, I was raising two daughters, working twenty hours a week and attaining scholarship grades in order to continue my studies. My life had become a recipe for disaster because I was straining and struggling without rest, relief or support. Depletion and exhaustion had become a way of life. My pain and emotions were so locked up inside they could only find expression through a burning pain in my right side.

Although I felt constant pain, I experienced acute agony if a man asked to take me out. If I felt attracted to anyone I would literally double over with pain. I didn't know how to deal with this somatic response, or even understand the fear that had become associated with men, so I lived in isolation, using great energy to contain and not allow any release of the suffering from my separation and divorce, or the difficulties of being on my own. I tried both a psychiatrist and group therapy, but both sessions made me feel sick to my stomach, so I quit going.

The pains in my side became worse. I didn't know what to do. I suffered several bouts of severe intestinal flu and took antibiotics, became more fatigued, then a sense of hopelessness overcame me. I felt completely alone except for my children. I felt as if I lived in a world that was without love. The burden of my life became too heavy to bear for the first time in all the years of struggling alone with the children, and I began to dream and long for death. As the thought of death overtook my mind, I began to believe that if I willed it, I could die. In my depressed and hopeless state, death seemed like the only way out of my situation.

I planned my departure well. I took the girls to Santa Monica beach. They would be happy playing on the beach and there would be people to care for them after I died. I already felt detached and I longed for release. The girls were full of life and when I settled them in with towels, food and toys, I told them I was going to take a long sleep and not to worry. I lay down and began a deep intense mantra of death. "God, take me, I am yours. God, take me now. I am dead." I repeated this over and over until it was my only thought and my only desire. I lost track of time, everything dissolved within. I thought I had died for I was no longer on the beach. I was in radiant light and all the burdens and loneliness were gone. I was with God in His great golden light of love.

Then I heard a voice. "Mommy, mommy. Someone is here."

I heard my girls' voices and felt the tugging of their little hands pulling me back to this world. "Oh, no," I thought, "I'm not dead." Slowly I came back into myself, but my body and my mind were at peace and I felt light and clear. I opened my eyes to the laughing smiles of my girls, and I was glad to see them. I reached out to hug them both in one embrace.

"Mommy, mommy. Look who's here," they both spoke together with excitement, trying to pull my head around.

As I turned around I looked into the brilliant blue eyes of a golden haired, bearded man, who was sitting behind me, watching over me with a kind, sweet smile.

"He was here all day while you were sleeping," they explained with excitement.

Then I noticed that it was dusk and nearly everyone was gone from the beach. I must have been out for hours. I felt so strange, so light–headed.

The stranger smiled and reassured me, saying "I was working this morning when I received an inner instruction that I was to come here, that there was someone who needed my help. I've been watching over you all day and taking care of your girls." And then he smiled shyly, and introduced himself, "My name is Ken."

I couldn't speak. I could only look, open eyed, into his eyes of light, which seemed as though they came from that glorious inner realm.

"Now it is time to go home. Come," he beckoned. While I took small steps to gain my balance, Ken gathered our things and put the girls into the back seat of his old station wagon. When I got in the front I noticed a large double bass musical instrument in the back.

"You can come back and get your car tomorrow," he suggested and I nodded in agreement. There was no way I could drive at that time because part of me was still in that place of light. How he knew I was on the beach was a mystery that could only be accepted, never explained. He was the manifestation of the love of God that I had connected with in my deep trance as I called out from the depths of my heart and soul. He had been sent to help me through this difficult time, a new friend, but also someone who seemed like a very old and dear friend.

"You're a musician?" I asked shyly as we drove along.

"Among other things," he smiled, and then we were silent the rest of the way home. Perhaps I had died. Everything seemed the same, but yet it was different. I was different, and he was here. The girls were awed by the mysterious happenings and this golden stranger.

From the beginning Ken was like he was part of the family, and he took charge in a natural easy way. He poured the bath and got the girls ready for bed. I stumbled around in the kitchen making sandwiches, feeling so strange, so new, so shy. The girls dropped off to sleep during his stories, and then he sat down and looked at me, and asked me what I thought I was doing on the beach.

I tried to talk, but only tears came. I let them flow. His tender glance allowed me to release my sorrow.

At last I could speak. "I wanted to die. I lay there and asked God to take me. He did. I thought I had died, but I came back."

"Why did you want to die?" he inquired gently.

"I've just had this feeling of hopelessness and depression. I feel so alone. Life is such a struggle. I didn't want to go on. I wanted to go back to God." I looked into his eyes, almost expecting him to laugh, but there was only respect and concern.

"Many of us want to go back to God, but we have to wait until He calls us home. We have to do our best until then."

I nodded, accepting this truth, the tears still gently flowing down my cheeks. I did not die that day, but I was given the gift of a friend who revealed truths that I had never imagined.

"God answered your prayers in one way, His way. He sent me to take care of you. I am here to help you, to help you want to live again."

Ken kept his word. He visited us every day, bringing fun, friendship and wisdom into our life, taking us to the beach, playing music for us, and sharing meals. I began to laugh and live again. When he took a carpentry job up in the Sierras and left us for a few weeks, we missed him, but all was well. I was busy with exams and the challenge of my responsibilities, but I had renewed energy and enthusiasm. I was enjoying my life again. I wanted to complete this year at college and then create a less stressful life.

About two weeks after Ken left I took a run on the beach. Suddenly I felt a pain on my chest and when I reached down I found a large lump on my right breast. I stopped running and began to shake with shock and fear. I could feel the lump and a pain in my right abdomen at the same time, and I knew there was something very wrong. I went home and made an appointment to see a doctor the next day. I was in shock and scared to death. Even though I took relaxing herbs that night I still couldn't sleep. I had never been so frightened. Up until then I had made a life style of fighting on my own, filling the days with responsibilities and hard work so that there was no time left to think. Now I was thinking and I didn't like my thoughts. All I saw was that I had gotten myself into a mess; I had pushed my body beyond endurance and now I had to pay the price.

The next day I sat on the table in the doctor's examination room and tried to look at the ceiling while he felt my breast. After a quick examination he turned to wash his hands, speaking with his back towards me as he said, "We'll have to operate right away. This is very big, could be serious. Can't lose any time. I'll have to have you sign this paper." The doctor was cold and brisk as he pushed the paper in front of me.

I started to read it. "What does this mean?" I said in a panic, fear like a knot in my chest and stomach.

"If we find it necessary, we'll remove the breast right then and there to save time and the risk of the cancer spreading."

"You want me to sign this so you can remove my breast? You mean I have cancer?" I questioned fearfully.

"Yes. We'll take a biopsy first to confirm everything, but it's always best to remove the breast right away."

"NEVER! I'll die first!" I shouted as I got up to leave.

"Where are you going? You'll die from this. What about your children? You can't go." I remembered the doctors who had bought sculptures from my art gallery, as they talked about how many operations it would take to buy a painting or a yacht. No one was going to buy something by taking off my breast. I felt angry as I turned my back on the doctor and walked out.

I walked hurriedly down the hall, refusing to answer either the doctor or his nurse who were calling after me, telling me not to leave. The L.A. summer heat and smog hit me like a brick wall. I was confused. I felt full of fear but there was some relief as I got into my own car, even though I was shaking from the shock. Finally I was able to drive home, but I didn't go back to school, and I didn't pick up the girls. I needed time to think. I wanted to be alone.

I lay in my small apartment watching the shadows of the leaves on my curtains, thinking about cancer, about dying, about my children. All the time I had been working and pushing and surviving and studying, this thing, this cancer, this lump had been growing. I saw it all, my refusal to release, to communicate and to let go of my emotional pain, and my refusal to face the physical pains that had been with me for some time. A few weeks before I had wanted to die, and now that I was actually faced with death, real death, I wanted to live. "I will live," I vowed. "I will find a way to get well."

The day went by. I sunk deeply into my self, watching the light and the leaves make patterns on the window blinds. I must have dozed off from exhaustion. When I woke, it was late afternoon. I would have to pick up the girls soon. The light was gold now and the leaves still. All the realities were still there, but there was no worry. I could have happily died at that moment, I felt so peaceful. From that peace one thought emerged, like a command, "Go and get that book you bought a couple of weeks ago. See what it says about cancer."

I got up slowly, in a daze. I remembered the book *Back to Eden* and went to get it. The cover had a picture of a man and women in a garden of tropical leaves. I'd been too busy to open it because of exams. There it was, on the bookshelf, waiting for me. I picked it up and it opened to a page in the center of the book where there was a picture of breast cancer. I began to read. I had to stop myself and go and get the girls, but as soon as I got home it was back to the book, holding it while making dinner, and reading it at the table. I stayed up most of the night, read the whole book and started again, making lists of what to buy and drawing up schedules. I was on fire. I had a plan and a direction, and I was going to make myself well.

I took my last exams, shopped for supplies, and started the treatment right away with a juice fast. My daily plan also included herbs, regular Epsom salt baths, enemas, and skin scrubbing. Very quickly I began to feel light, clear and empty. Energy increased, as did a feeling of joy and excitement. Exams were over so I was free to concentrate completely on my healing.

I realized I needed help, and the only person I could ask was Ken. He was in the Sierras, at Mammouth, camped out somewhere, but I knew he went to Hot Creek at night to bathe in the pools. I would find him. He would help me. I realized that my death wish had manifested in my body. Ken had helped me cure my longing for death and I knew he would help me heal what I had created in my body.

I got up at five in the morning, carried the girls outside and laid them onto a bed of pillows and blankets in the back seat of my old VW. They slept as I drove north through the cool morning hours so we could miss the worst of the desert heat. They were still sleeping when we drove by the sign announcing Death Valley, and I laughed. Life or death. That was what it had come down to. I was ready to fight death for my life.

We arrived in Mammouth about noon. I drove through the town a couple of times and then reality hit me. How would we find him? Where would we stay? I didn't know anyone. I felt scared, but I hid it from the girls.

"Mommy, can we have an ice cream cone?" Glad for something to do, I parked in a shopping center. We all got cones and sat on the grass. I wondered how I would find him? Just then I noticed his car pulling up to the stop light. He had found us again.

"Ken, Ken, here we are." I got up, yelling and waving. He looked around and saw us and drove over, and we all hugged each other with happiness and relief.

"What are you doing here?" He searched my eyes, and saw the depths. "OK, we'll talk about it later. I'll take you to my campsite. I see you've got your sleeping bags," he smiled. "I've got a really great campsite in the woods."

We followed him outside of town where he had pitched his tent. I never could have found him; that's why divine providence had arranged it for us. We set up our tent, ate some watermelon and then set off for Hot Creek.

"Sure is funny. I left work early. Never usually come into town till after dark," he said as his eyes twinkled with the mystery of it all. I was happy to be with him again.

While the kids swam and played, I told him the news. He sat quietly, watching my face, taking it all in. Then I was quiet, holding silent questions just under the surface, scared, shaking inside, trembling outside. Now that I was faced with death I wanted to live. I wanted to raise my girls and do my best in this life. I let the tears flow with the stream going by, absorbing the sound of its movement as it calmed my mind. Ken was silent for a long time.

Finally he spoke, "Body isn't much different than the mind. It just takes longer to clear. You have a lesson to learn here. I'm glad you came. Let's see what we can do, but now, its time to swim."

Hot Creek was wonderful. Great bubbling bursts of hot water came up from under rocks on one side of the creek, while cold fresh quick water flowed by on the other. Hot and cold. Hot and cold. We swam from the bubbling heat to the cold rush of the stream. There were warm and quiet shallows and pools we floated to further along the mossy green banks. We played, and swam, got hot, came out, rested, cooled down and then returned to do it all over again. The cycles of playing and soaking made me feel clean and clear and light. Then a great grey cloud swirled overhead and hail came down. We laughed as we tried to escape the pounding from the dramatic thunderstorm sky. Finally, as dusk settled we dressed and drove back to the campsite, feeling drowsy, clean, soft and warm. The girls fell asleep and had to be carried into our tent.

Ken and I talked a while. Then he practiced some of the mantras and spiritual healings he had used on me before. As his hands moved above my aura, we repeated the prayers of protection out loud. His hands stopped again and again over my right colon where I had the pain. There was darkness there, a shadow of negativity that seemed connected to and even more of a problem than the breast lump. The breast lump seemed more of a symptom than the real cause. I went to sleep repeating the prayer of protection and healing that he taught me, feeling safe, feeling loved, feeling taken care of.

The days sped by. I fasted, did enemas, took herbs, practiced yoga and breathing, and spent the days at the hot spring, and then when Ken joined us there after work he gave me shiatsu and reflexology treatments, taught me tai chi and meditation, played music, and practiced his healing mantras. Within a few days I began to feel incredibly well.

During one treatment he put his hand on my breast lump. "Now imagine pure white light and love are coming from above through me, into my hand, then into your breast. Imagine that this light and love is dissolving the lump, turning the darkness into light."

I went with the vision, feeling the energy moving through my body, feeling the lump dissolve, becoming light and love and peace, lifted up out of my body into another dimension. I knew God was healing me.

When I came back to myself I was lying quietly in my sleeping bag. Again, a death. Again, a rebirth. I felt my breast. The lump was gone. "Ken. Ken, the lump is gone." I shouted to him.

"I know" his voice whispered sleepily from his tent. "Sweet dreams."

When I woke in the morning the lump was back, but it was softer and less painful. "The lump is back, Ken, it's back."

"Only temporarily. You still have lessons to learn," he reassured me.

The golden summer days sped by. I was healing. I was going to be well. We were creating a new world of healing and happiness, a world of purity, beauty and spirituality. I was a child of God. I trusted. I surrendered. I believed. I was clay being molded for a new way of life. Innocence had returned.

One evening Ken asked me to lie on a blanket under the stars, and then he picked up his saxophone and told me he was going to send the music into the areas of my ascending colon where the darkness had come from. He began to play and I felt the music come into my being and lift me up and out of my body. So light. So free. So pure. I became the body that is not this body, but a finer body in another dimension beyond the physical, where transformation and healing take place. When I returned to my physical body the darkness in the colon area had decreased.

I fasted days on orange juice followed by days on watermelon. I was thin and clean and well. I took herbal enemas, drank Red Clover herb tea, and took capsules of Golden Seal, Cayenne, and Saw Palmetto. I lost the desire for food. Life took on radiance, joy and happiness beyond measure. When I watched Ken practice tai chi I could actually see the light streaming from his hands creating golden pathways in the air.

Before a month had gone by the breast lump disappeared, and the pain in my colon was gone. I was more myself than I had ever been. I had returned to the innocence of childhood trust where there were no worries, fears or hurts. My life was golden with light because I was filled with trust, love and faith.

The summer came to an end. We had to return to Santa Monica where I was supposed to go back to college. The girls had to return to school. I felt my fear returning. I didn't want to go. I didn't want this beautiful time to end.

"Times like this can't last forever. You have been given healing, a new body. This gift is to be shared," Ken explained. I tried to hear, but I felt as though my heart was breaking. "You can't hold on. You have to move with the changes," he insisted.

We packed both our cars and headed south, down through the desert, the mountains on the right, Death Valley now on the left, and then over the pass into L.A. Santa Monica was busy, hot, dusty, and the sky was grey with smog. My apartment was cool and restful after the journey, but my body felt tight and tense for the first time all summer. Ken left to visit with his parents, and I faced the reality of returning to the old shell of my life. I wondered if I could live here again, if I could find a way to face this loneliness and this struggle. Could I do it?

Over the next few days the girls went back to school, and I returned to college to sign up for classes. I felt strange, like I didn't belong. All the excitement and love of learning was gone. The academic life seemed empty in comparison to the profound healing of body and soul I had experienced in the mountains.

When Ken came to visit I felt a deep change in him. He was very quiet. I felt frightened because I sensed what he was going to say. Finally, after dinner when the kids had gone to bed, he shared his news. "I have to go to Hawaii. I have a friend there that needs me. It's time for me to move on. You are strong and well now. You have to live your own life."

My heart raced from fear. I could hardly breathe. I wondered how he could leave? It was then I realized that I had fallen in love with him. Somehow I imagined that we would always be together. We had been so busy with my healing and the beauty of the time in the mountains that we had never explored the possibility of our being together as man and woman.

"I thought you would stay with us. I thought we were meant to be together," I stammered and blushed.

"Only for a time. My work with you is finished."

I began to cry as I confessed "I don't want to be well if that means you have to leave." He held me and let me cry, and when he said goodnight, I knew it would be a long time before I saw him again.

I faced loneliness again, and it seemed worse after the fullness of friendship, love and support. I couldn't go back to my old ways. If I had to raise my girls alone, I had to find a better way. I had to find a way to live a spiritual life and still face my responsibilities. Registration day came and went at the college, but I lay day after day in my apartment watching the light and the leaves change as the hours crept by. I couldn't return to my former life, but I didn't see any doors opening. I had a new body and a new self. Where was I to go and what was I to do?

After the registration deadline passed, I went to my college to tell my counselor I was dropping out of school when I bumped into my yoga teacher. He invited me to a seminar they were having that weekend. Yogi Bhajan was coming. I grasped at straws, got a babysitter and went along. I had to find a spiritual way of life. Before the weekend was over I had agreed to live in the Tucson ashram and help start a program for the children there. I couldn't wait to leave L.A. We had a garage sale, sold everything except what we could fit in the VW, and the girls and I and set off into the desert.

My time in the Tucson ashram was woven of rich growth and hard lessons. Community devotions began at 3 a.m. when we were awakened by flute music and cups of tea borne by white robed, turbaned brothers. After three hours of yoga, mantras and singing, we raised the ashram flag at 6 a.m. when the already burning September sun was urging the day to begin. Our daily schedule included karma yoga, singing, devotions, meals, and serving the poor in the free soup kitchen. There was laughter and song, games and fun, gardening, yoga, music, and sunshine, but also tears. I purchased a large tent so the girls and I could have our own space in the garden. The hot summer faded into autumn. The life of yoga and service strengthened us, and when we returned to L.A just before Christmas, poorer, wiser and homeless, I had become a yoga teacher and had gained experience and knowledge in natural living and healing. This helped me to create a positive foundation for the next cycle of my life.

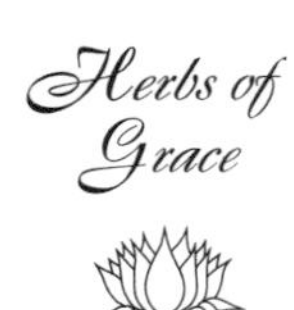

Miraculously, I got my old apartment back. However, once again the setting was the same, but the reality was different. We had sold everything, so we lived simply and the situation felt temporary. I had car and money troubles, but work opened up in a health and beauty spa in Westwood, and soon we were back on our feet again. The girls returned to school and life went on again. I never regretted leaving college because I was deep in my own study of healing and working with massage, reflexology and yoga every day at the spa.

I connected with women at the day care center in Santa Monica and we began to take camping trips to the hot springs in the valley over the saddle mountain behind Santa Barbara. Between us we had a total of eight children and it was a merry group that would drive out in a large van on Friday night and spend our weekend soaking, sunning, exchanging massages, hiking and doing yoga. I joined a Gestalt group once a week and the sessions helped me to identify and clear feelings and emotions, as well as take responsibility for them. I also learned Esalen massage that took me beyond the limitation of time into a dance of graceful inner light and sensitivity. My previous life of isolation was now opening up to love and friendship. There was still a strong deep urge to leave Los Angeles, but no clear direction.

Most of my women friends danced with Emily Conrad at her Continuum classes early in the morning near downtown L.A. At 6 a.m. I joined the class to celebrate the Three Gong Ceremony and release the kundalini serpent of creativity. At that time her movement classes began with breathing and undulations until the energy moved to raise the body *'up from the dead.'* Once we reached an upright position we explored diving into the unconscious, curling and uncurling the spine as we dove forward, slowly, so slowly that it seemed that we were diving endlessly into inner feeling space. When this movement was complete we explored the wings of the *Caduceus*, the serpentine curling through the chakras that releases in flight. These movements caused my spirit to soar and my body undulated with the movements of winged flight towards the end of each class.

Our women's group also met regularly every week at each others' homes to explore the issues of femininity. We found support and love as we bared the bones of our emotions and minds, releasing our repressions, pain, anger, hurt and longings. It was special for me to experience the beauty, grace and intelligence of each woman in our group. We had all suffered, experienced divorce and were raising our children on our own, but we had the opportunity to be true to our inner selves and explore healing, spirituality and femininity in a way that women more protected and sheltered by husband and home could not imagine. We were discovering our wellsprings of inner strength and sharing strength, support and resources with each other. Above all we were recognizing that we could create meaningful, creative and beautiful lives on our own as we learned to overcome our hardships.

SHASTA FLOWER

This group support helped me to develop new levels of inner strength and gave me the courage to take a long journey the following summer of 1973 when my children and I drove to Canada to visit family in Vancouver, British Columbia. On the way back we stopped off to visit my cousin in Mount Shasta and loved the area so much we decided to stay. During my time there, I became deeply involved in visiting local spiritual teachers, Pearl, Stan and Thaedra. Although we lived separately, the Mount Shasta community provided opportunities to live the role of a lay healer, sharing herbs, vegetarian wholefood diets and healing with the other women and children. I practiced affirmations, visualizations and color healing. It was an exciting time for me as I sharpened my mind through the focus of seeking light and truth. My self–healing continued with purification fasts, meditation, and the creation of large cloth mandalas to externalize my visions and harmonize the evolution taking place between my mental, emotional and physical bodies.

During these early years herbs became a larger and larger part of my life, as the health and healing movement took hold in California. Our group shared, discovered, explored and supported each other as we created a new health and wholefood lifestyle. As the community expanded and needs grew, we formed a food co–operative, a health and wholefood shop, and then a vegetarian restaurant. We felt we were riding the wave of creative, exciting changes as the culture grew up around us offering healing centers, books, magazines, seminars, women's groups and herbal gatherings. Our favorite herbal tea blends became packaged products in colorful boxes. Yoga, spiritual teachings, sufi dancing, massage and other communities beckoned to us to include them in our lives. We supported and gave service to each other as we created our new vision of community and found new ways to earn our living.

I loved my pantry filled with jars of herbs, grains, nuts, seeds, dried fruits and herbs. These supplies formed the core of the natural vegetarian, wholefood diet we were exploring. Cookbooks began coming out and we all swapped recipes and ideas. It was great fun, learning, creating and sharing together.

My own self–healing continued on new levels during this time. On the psychological level I reached through the fears of my shy nature, opening to warm companionship as I felt more secure. I also began to communicate my inner life as I met people who were more loving and receptive, rather than holding it all inside and living in fear and isolation.

On the physical level I continued with the herbs, juices, raw foods and a wholesome vegetarian diet, healing any illness with natural methods. Three times a week I took an Epsom salts bath, scrubbed and oiled my body and did a thorough foot reflexology treatment. Gradually the crystals and painful areas in my feet lessened until the last one on the spleen reflex area surfaced in a spell of itching, a healing crisis that eventually receded. Deep levels of toxins surfaced, requiring attention and all the symptoms were healed through self–applied herbs and

natural medicine home treatments. I drove two hundred miles south each week to Paradise, near Chico, for a series of chiropractic adjustments. As my lower back straightened I became stronger and more direct in other aspects of my life. My digestion also improved.

During this time my spiritual centers awakened and I received dreams that guided me with visions, teachings and images that nourished me with love. Morning after morning I would awake in bliss, striving to capture the memory of some incredibly beautiful landscape and faces full of love and light. In one dream I travelled to a school in some realm of existence where I spent the night looking through magnificent golden books where the mysteries of life were explained to me. Another night I was in a healing temple surrounded by columns and robed figures who gave me a new spine and nervous system. Another time I went inside Mount Shasta with great beings of light, and later Pearl told me in person that she had seen me there. I didn't remember many details of that dream experience, but the thought of it filled me with radiant happiness. Once when my twelve year old son, Galon, went up the mountain on a camping expedition he got caught in a storm. All through that night I protected him in my dream with my arms while great demons tried to frighten and hurt him. When I awoke, I drove up the mountain and met him as he arrived in Panther Meadow, still shaken from his experience, but alright. I didn't tell him about my dream right away but instead let him tell me about the storm, how it blew their tent away and how they had to hold on to a rock to avoid being blown over the cliff. When I told him about the dream we were amazed together as we held each other with relief and happiness, glad that he was safe, and knowing that God had been with both of us.

About the time that my life was opening to the light my new teachers were helping to awaken in me, a woman in Dunsmuir began to slander and persecute me. She had harbored a vengeful jealousy well hidden by a seeming friendship until she couldn't control her feelings any more. Although she had attained a high level of expertise in the Rosicrucian path, her energies had moved to the dark side and night after night I awakened to sense her purposeful negative energy focused on me. Then one night the energy seemed like a knife entering me, and even with my eyes closed I could picture her sitting on her own bed, on the other side of the river, projecting darkness that entered into the weak place on the right side, the area I thought I had healed with Ken in the Sierras. Although I felt weak, I forced myself to get up, put the children in the car in the middle of the night, and drive until I was free of her telepathic hate. I didn't stop driving until I reached Ashland, Oregon, and then I joined the children in the back of the van for some restless sleep. In the morning I went into the metaphysical bookstore and discussed the experience with the owners. They told me to talk to my spiritual teachers and assured me that I would be protected if I asked for help.

Eventually I sought the help of Pearl and Stan, renowned Mt. Shasta spiritual leaders, who gave me treatments and affirmations, helping me to protect myself, and assuring me that eventually the energy she was releasing would return to her. Each day I practiced meditations and visualizations and created healing mandalas as I fought the dark energies of this woman's hateful jealousy. They told me they had been aware of her dark influence on the young people who came seeking teachers and they assured me this opportunity was a way to break her false image and destroy her power over others. Although I couldn't understand why she had chosen to

attack me, I did the work my teachers instructed me to do to protect myself and ward off her dark and vengeful energy.

The final healing came one night as I finished a hand–stitched velvet mandala I had been working on for weeks. It was a circular view of the chakras, the smallest earth chakra like the center of a flower, within all the expanding flower chakras, circled at the outer edge with hundreds of gold leaves representing the crown chakra. I was putting the gold leaves on one evening when the pain in my right side became very strong. I knew she was focused on hurting me again, but my reaction was different this time. Instead of wanting to run away I became angry. That was a rare feeling for me but I decided I had had enough. I was going to end this persecution then and there, so I lay down on my bed so that I could look at the mandala on the wall. I imagined myself inside the six foot chakra flower with the gold leaves all around me, symbolic of my golden aura. Once I had placed myself mentally inside this protection I closed my eyes and began the mantra, "God is healing me. I am being healed," over and over, hundreds of times, with full concentration, until I became the mantra and disappeared into divine light.

When I came back to normal consciousness, my body was vibrating with gentle undulations. I felt light, love and energy pouring into me from the crown chakra on the top of my head, and moving down throughout my entire body. An exquisite flow of brilliant, energetic, electric nourishment filled my being with pulsing light and energy. After some time this flow of undulations gently subsided and I lay in a state of bliss until dawn, knowing that some great change had been made, and knowing once more that when the call is made with one's entire being the answer comes greater than one can even imagine. Tears flowed gently down my cheeks, tears of happiness, of love and gratitude. More and more I was discovering how much love pervaded everything, and that we only need to open ourselves to receive this love. I knew without any doubt that we only need to ask with our full being and that we will be answered with love.

The next day I felt a pain in my side like dry ice that slowly began to move down my leg. Over a period of three days it descended. I couldn't walk, so I soaked my feet in Epsom salts which drew the pain down over a period of three days. When the pain reached my right foot it became swollen and sensitive. I was still in a state of joy and bliss and knew that negativity was leaving and that I was being protected and supported through this process, so I never experienced any fear or uncertainty. My being was filled with radiance. I was being healed by the forces of love and light and I was surrendering with full joy.

After this experience I no longer felt any negative energy from this woman, and a short time later her land was flooded during a winter storm. Water destroyed her sheds and a mobile home and washed the driveway into the river. A few months later her home was burned to the ground and all her possessions were destroyed. I heard that she narrowly escaped with her life. My spiritual teachers told me that this natural elemental vengeance was the result of her own darkness returning to her.

During this period I read Castenada's *Journey to Ixtlan*, absorbing the teachings concerning the worthy opponent. I realized I had survived and emerged victorious from an initiation and rejoiced that I was supported to walk the path of love and light because I had refused to enter into a war with her on her terms. My teachers guided me to reach higher levels of spirituality which protected me against her negativity. In my heart and mind I transmitted compassionate love toward her and also thanked her for providing the resistance which gave me the opportunity to progress on my spiritual path. She left the area for a while and when she returned she did not have the same powerful influence over others, nor was she able to fool young people into believing that she was a spiritual teacher. My teachers had told me in the early days of my difficulties with her that her mirror of credibility would be broken when she used her powers to hurt someone, and this proved true.

With this trial behind me life moved on. Spring was in the air and life was full with children, friends and healing. New friends moved into the area and the community continued to expand, bringing excitement and joy as well as new challenges.

During the 1974 summer holidays all three of my children came down with chickenpox. When I called the doctor and asked him what I should do, he replied, "Nothing." "What do you mean, nothing?" I countered, annoyed. When he replied "You just have to wait and let it run its course," I realized that he didn't know anything about relieving illness so I consulted my healing bible *Back to Eden*.

My eldest daughter, Casel, came down with the chickenpox first, and true to her nature she suffered silently, keeping very still while her body developed pustules and the fever raged. I applied poultices of Golden Seal and Comfrey to her swollen glands, and made a paste of Golden Seal and vitamin E oil to put on each pustule. I served her endless cups of herb teas to cleanse her system and reduce the fever. The period of discomfort was short and she was soon running about again. Regular applications of almond oil, wheat germ oil and Chickweed herbal baths reduced the itching and prevented scarring as the pustules dried and healed.

Just as Casel was recovering, my youngest daughter, Chalice, came down with the chickenpox. True to her nature, she made a big fuss, moaned and groaned and demanded constant attention. However, as her pustules were only on her scalp, under her hair, I kept her head covered in a mess of poultice herbs and wrapped it in a turban. Her fever and discomfort abated quickly without any complications or weakness.

My son, Galon, came down with the symptoms last. He manifested a few, very large pustules on his shoulders and back. His period of discomfort lasted only one night and a day and my ministrations, tried and proven by now, minimized the effects of the chicken pox. When I later saw how long and how much other children suffered during that epidemic and how bad their scarring was, I considered myself fortunate to have had the herbs at hand and to have known how to use them.

Our Mount Shasta and Dunsmuir communities were warm and rich with exchange as we shared knowledge and supported each other. Each health crisis manifested a support system, a team effort that gradually built a body of knowledge and experience. The women gained trust in their inner intuition and strength to overcome health problems, instead of seeking quick remedies and radical treatment from the medical profession. We gloried in sharing our tales of success and our children blossomed under our natural nurturing, willing participants in the creation of a new way. There was a wonderful feeling of sharing. We knew we were not alone in any crisis. I absorbed the community spirit after so many years of isolation in Los Angeles. Anyone's illness became a community problem and we all contributed to the nursing. Natural medicine became a focus for loving, caring and sharing. Although our children still caught colds, flus and fevers and suffered from gastrointestinal troubles, we found the symptoms did not last long, discomfort was not as great, and recovery was a positive return to health. When treatment included a light diet or fasting, herbs, baths, reflexology and poultices, the return to daily life was quick, clean and clear. After the herbs, diets and treatments we felt better and returned to work and play, instead of taking days or weeks to feel like ourselves again.

We spoke about herbs as though they were our friends. Herbs became an important part of our lives and we were comforted knowing that we could contribute meaningful treatment and natural nursing for our family and friends when they were ill or injured. Now, whenever I think of Golden Seal I remember the chickenpox epidemic, septic wounds or infections. Using herbs in daily life experience creates a relationship that is steeped in personal wisdom and experience. This is the best and deepest training.

Rainbow Flower

Two years later my experience at Mount Shasta seemed complete, so we headed south, visiting hot springs and healing centers until we reached the Palm Springs area where we wanted to stay for the winter. The desert took a strong hold on me. I loved the simplicity, the clarity, the hazy violet mountains, and the rainbow–filled sky over Whitewater tucked between desert hills, west of Desert Hot Springs. The air felt clean and dry, the sun shone every day, rainshowers freshened the air with the fragrance of Chaparral. The girls loved the hot springs. We went swimming every day after they got out of school. I got a job managing a health and beauty spa in Palm Springs and soon I was deeply involved in reorganizing the treatments, training the staff and learning shiatsu from the owner and his staff from Japan. The spa doubled its income due to my management and I experienced great satisfaction from the success.

When women came into the spa draped in gold chains, jewelled rings, earrings and bracelets, I asked them to remove them with newfound confidence. During their massages, these wealthy but troubled women talked about their lives. Counselling became an important part of my work. I learned that wealth, husbands, and status in no way immunize us from internal suffering. I had my first experience of being independently capable, and the sense of accomplishment gave me new strength. I began to recognize my own worth because these women appreciated me, my work and the contribution I made to their lives.

As early as 1975 I developed fresh Aloe Vera facials and body wraps to treat sunburn. Although Aloe Vera is a well–known product today, at that time the packs were revolutionary,

especially in a luxury hotel. When clients suffered from hangovers we wrapped them up in cloths that had been soaked in herbal brews. The detoxification process relieved their symptoms and released excess weight and water. I blended natural beauty facials individually, using fresh fruit, herbs, Aloe Vera, vitamin E, and honey. I also brought in fresh beauty products from the Golden Door, created by Edmund Bordeaux Szekeley, translator of the Dead Sea Scrolls and author of *The Essene Gospel of Peace*. Massage treatments included Swedish massage, Shiatsu and Reflexology. The results spoke for themselves. Clients returned again and again during their stay and soon guests arrived at the hotel ready to schedule treatments, having heard about them from their friends. At the end of the season the management told me that my efforts resulted in the most profitable and successful spa season ever and they asked me to return. For the first time in years I had made good money and I was pleased to continue.

It was June and unbearably hot. When the girls got out of school we headed for the ocean in our van, but our first stop was a bluegrass festival on Mount San Jacinto above Palm Springs. The crowds were lively and as we wandered around, enjoying the music, I noticed a group of long–haired desert people selling airbrushed clothes by an airbrushed car that was painted with roses, rainbows and angels. I was drawn irresistibly toward their joy and laughter. They appeared radiantly healthy as they danced and sang and bargained their rainbow painted clothes. The girls and I were captivated and enchanted with their happy energy when one brother noticed us and approached.

After introducing himself as Michael, he told us that they were the Rainbow Family and that they lived about an hour away in a commune in the desert, near Warner Hot Springs where they practiced the Essene way of life and painted 'rainbows' (that's what he called their clothes) for a living.

"Hey, we're having a festival. Starts tomorrow. Yer invited."

The girls were jumping up and down with excitement, "Please, please, mommy, let's go."

"Do ya have wheels?" he enquired, and when I nodded, he danced around us, "Primo. Far out! Follow us to the ranch. We're outa here. Go git your wheels."

That invitation made us so excited we ran all the way back to the van and were back within minutes. Michael introduced us to the group and soon we were heading south. I knew I was going somewhere I had always wanted to go. Through Szekeley, I knew the Essenes were called 'the pure people,' and that they practiced purification as a way of life. When we drove through the gates on the triangle of land bordered on all sides by national forest preserve I knew instinctively I was home. I did not pass back through those gates for nearly two months, so deeply did I enter into the life there. I soon realized that everything I had experienced until that time had been a preparation for this next step, and I knew I was ready for transformation.

The community was generous, and soon the girls and I were dressed in 'rainbows' and living in a tipi. As the days sped swiftly by, I learned to make delicious raw food salads, sun tea and biblical bread. I also learned how to walk at night with my eyes closed, to dance, to sing. After a period of apprenticeship in the studio, cleaning the equipment and watching, I learned how to paint rainbow teeshirts, following the stencils that Michael made, painting one ray of rainbow color after another.

We merged into the lifestyle with ease, feeling completely at home. I wanted to shine like them, to be light like them, to laugh like them. Soon, all my excess weight fell off and I could run like a deer and accomplish every yoga pose that had resisted me before. I went on a long fast, first on grape juice, then on water. After the morning work I climbed up the hill and stood on a rock, faced the wind, dancing mudras and breathing in the ecstasy of life. The entire universe seemed as if it were woven of light–filled energy.

Every night and every morning someone would stoke up the sauna fire. Inside the hot wooden room we scrubbed each other with stiff brushes, hit ourselves with eucalyptus branches, and then ran under the cold water shower. When all the women gathered into sister saunas we honored our femininity, celebrated our wisdom and our heartspace with each other. When we needed to cool down we ran down the dirt road, naked under the stars, singing and laughing, celebrating joy and freedom, like nymphs, and howling to the coyotes in the night desert.

It was an even deeper level of sisterhood than I experienced in Mount Shasta, because there in the desert wilderness we could commune with nature, the earth, the sky, the sun, moon, stars and plants, and find in their reflection our own mother nature within. We all represented different aspects of the feminine. We were sisters, but we were also teachers for each other. Meadow taught me to be still, to sit waiting under a tree or on a rock and to listen to the sacred sounds of nature. Lisa taught me the warrior space of strength and endurance in the garden and on the building projects. Crystal shared the delicate skills of beadwork, stitchery and Mexican eyes–of–God, and Karen revealed the mysteries of herbs, raw food salads, sun tea and biblical bread. I contributed my motherhood nurturing experiences, and my dances, clothes designs and healing skills.

After this two–month retreat the community asked me to go to a fair in Palm Springs to sell rainbows. I didn't want to return to the outside world, but Michael said he would go with me and be my guide. Heading north in the rainbow car, we flew over the desert. Being away from the commune made me realize that I was seeing the sky and the earth like never before. My vision was clear and perfect. Since twelve years of age I had worn glasses and had limited blurry vision because of astigmatism, but now as I watched birds move, noticing every nuance of every movement, I realized my vision had been healed by the herbs, fasting and raw food diet. Clouds held enchanted worlds of shape, form and vision. I felt as if I were seeing for the first time in my life. Everything was crystal clear and radiantly beautiful.

From the mountain overlooking the desert valley, Palm Springs, the green jewel of the desert, beckoned to us when we stopped the car before descending into civilization. I had become one of the Rainbow Family, golden, shining, light and pure, and we were here to bring our message of radiant health and joy to the people at the fair. Now I was the one selling rainbows in front of the rainbow car, dancing the joy of the bargaining, making jokes and moving to the music of the tapes.

The next day Michael said he had a surprise for me. "We're going to take a hike. I want to show you a primo nectar place."

We bought four mangoes at the health food store and drove to one of the Indian canyons southwest of Palm Springs. After parking the car we headed up a trail until we heard the sound

of a waterfall. Laughing with delight we entered the most exquisite oasis, where water surrounded a great rounded stone which rose up from the centre of the pool as though reaching up to the water falling all over it from above. I sensed it was a sacred place and we both felt awed that we should have the good fortune to be here by ourselves. After a few moments of respectful reflection, we became aware once again that we were hot and dusty, so we quickly threw off our clothes and dove into the pool. After refreshing ourselves in the cool water, Michael handed me two of the mangoes, and holding one mango in each hand, we swam out to the rounded stone and climbed up. Hunched in the spray, covered with glistening drops, water rainbows between us and the sun, we devoured the mangoes. Then, diving into the water and climbing back up again, we played and swam until, exhausted, all we could do was lie on hot rocks until the burning sun sent us back to the water to laugh and play again. When we heard voices we collected our belongings and slipped quietly back down the trail, leaving the sacred space for the next visitors. On that day I experienced the pure magic of primitive children celebrating the joy of nature, one of the most beautiful experiences of my life. It was amazing to see how each step of the way we are prepared for the next experience. Two months before, I never could have laughed and swum, climbed up on the stone again and again, and dove into the water with such light freedom. My body had become clean and strong, like when I was a child.

Back at the Rainbow Ranch we were deep in the heat of full summer, and had to remain inside at midday. It became too hot to paint. We began to take short trips out in the morning and afternoon to ponds and streams to keep cool, and we jumped over the fence after midnight into Warner Hot Springs pool to swim and play until dawn.

During the third month of my stay I began a purification program of fasting, herbs and raw food. After about thirty days on this program boils began to appear, first on my right knee, then on my left thumb where I lost my nail. I intensified the purifying herb teas and enemas, but large boils appeared under my right arm, draining off the poison from my breast lump, so I trusted the process and allowed it to continue. The boils were incredibly painful, intensifying just before they burst. One after another they came, nine in all from my right underarm, and then after one last boil on my chin, they ceased. I was amazed to experience how deep purification could release toxins long after we believe we have been healed.

Spiritual Sun Flower

My healing was complete just as summer turned into autumn. It was now time for me to return to Palm Springs, the Spa and the winter season. I thought I had felt light after my healing in the Sierras, but this healing had taken me to a new level and I realized I was moving forward in my spiritual journey. I knew that I was being drawn toward a way of life that would serve my highest purpose. Instead of feeling only the suffering of the world, I lived a dance of energy, joy and light.

Because of the deep purification I became open to receive nourishment from higher and subtler energies. I had released, let go, and created space that was now being filled with a new life and a higher way of being.

My new self was soon put to the test as I returned to work at the Palm Springs spa for the 1975 winter season. My new management position included further responsibilities and my life as a healer took on new dimensions. Continuing the momentum of five months of physical purification I began to repeat spiritual and mental affirmations received from Pearl in Mount Shasta. During my hourly drive from Desert Hot Springs across the valley to the Canyon Golf and Racquet Resort and home again, drinking in the beauty of the wide blue skies and violet mountains, I repeated again and again, "I am the temple of the living God." I felt sacred, like a temple, open, ready to receive the spirit and the purity that I sought. My heart, voice and soul called out the affirmations again and again.

As if in answer to my call I met satsangis from the Radha Soami (Lord of the Soul) path of meditation, who were disciples of the living master, Maharaj Charan Singh Ji. This spiritual path had come to my attention several times during the past year. I was already living three of their vows, complete vegetarianism, the moral life, and abstinence from alcohol and drugs, but the vow to do two and one–half hours of meditation daily seemed quite impossible. After I hired two satsangis to work with me at the spa, met others and attended a satsang, I began to feel that if others could meditate, I could too. From the moment I walked in the satsang room and felt the presence of the Master I felt that I was home. During the winter I prepared for initiation by reading the required books and following all the vows for three months.

I was initiated in May 1976 and began the practice of meditation to purify my mind, emotions and body as a preparation for the release of the soul from mind and body at death. I felt as though I had been longing for this path all my life. As a child in Sunday school and later in church I longed to be with Christ, a living son of God, and used to ask the teachers where I could go to be with Him. This wish was finally fulfilled when I travelled to London, England, in June, 1976 to attend satsang with the Master. His light and love and radiance were all and more than I had ever dreamed of, and my life rejoiced in gratitude that this longing had at last been answered.

After I returned from London, the spa closed for the summer and I traveled north to visit my family in Canada. I worked the remainder of the summer in a hot springs outside San Luis Obispo in California. It was the perfect place to spend our summer vacation. The children swam and played all day while I worked nearby in the spa, giving massage, facials, shiatsu and reflexology treatments. I also studied Iridology and the Bach flower remedies in the evening. My daily practice of meditation calmed my mind and uplifted my spirit. Finally, my life seemed full and good on all levels. I now understood that the struggle of life was a spiritual exercise. I realized that the universe and divine forces had supported me in a direct way throughout all the years, and that valuable tools had been given to help me live my life and attain my highest goals.

I was committed to the Palm Springs spa for another season, yet every time the thought entered my mind I had the feeling I wasn't going back. I didn't know where else I was supposed to be, so at the end of August I returned to the desert and settled in an apartment. I was early for

the spa season, so I attended a Polarity Seminar with Pierre Pannetier. One night, later that week, I was swimming in the Desert Hot Springs spa with my children when I had a vision of myself at Healing Waters in Eden, Arizona – a center I had visited in February with some of my old Rainbow family friends. The vision was very clear. The next day I received a letter. My friend, Michael had moved there and he was sending me a complimentary invitation to attend an Iridology and Herbology seminar with Dr. Raymond Christopher. He also extended an invitation for me to join their community if I wanted to stay.

Call it synchronicity, call it craziness, call it courage or destiny, whatever, but within two days I had packed everything and we were driving east to Arizona. The risk was enormous, but my instinct said to go for it, so I did. I knew the women I had trained at the spa would be able to run the place if I didn't return.

The children were always ready for an adventure and as it turned out that's what we got. When we left Palm Springs, heading east on the highway, we drove under an immense and brilliant rainbow that seemed like a doorway welcoming us to a new life. On the pass between California and Arizona we ran into a storm. All night we drove through torrential rain, lightning and thunder; it was like driving through a light show. In the early morning hours we left Phoenix and the storm behind. Alone on the road we flew up into the hills beneath a quiet starry sky. When we pulled into Healing Waters at dawn, the sky was clear and bright. The girls were asleep in the station wagon, so I climbed the little hill and took a good long soak in the source hot pool, treasuring the delicate dawn mist and my solitude beneath the fading stars in the rosy sky. When I walked down into the community I saw a sweat lodge fire burning. Michael must be there, I thought with a grin. That brother was always purifying.

Sure enough as I walked up to the fire, I saw him hunched over, wrapped in a blanket. I hunched over too and sat beside him for a a while before he noticed me. Then with a laugh my old friend leapt up to welcome me and introduce me to the others. Some of the brothers had visited the Rainbow Family ranch so we nodded, reconnecting, beginning community again.

The sweat lodge was hot and high, causing the spirit to open as the body melted. The prayers we spoke and sang from our hearts united us in loving community. An hour later we crawled out into the day, steaming in the misty dawn, and dove into the swimming pool to cool ourselves, and laugh and play like young children, our bodies light and free. What a beautiful way to begin my new life here.

The community was dedicated to creating a healing center and before the day was out I had met old and new friends. The children and I were given a room in the old Victorian hotel and I received karma yoga duties to care for Dr. Christopher as well as to help out in the kitchen and the healing room. I was amazed and happy as my life unfolded in my new home. I felt glad to be living in a community again, because as much as I had enjoyed my life and work in Palm Springs it had been difficult to both work and care for my children without any help.

I was completely ready in body, mind and spirit to receive all Dr. Christopher had to offer. I had experienced enough with my own healing to recognize the truth he shared with us that was drawn from his years of experience. His sweetness and noble character reminded me of my spiritual teacher, and his crop of white hair shone like a crown of wisdom.

Time and again we witnessed his harmonious consciousness. He was a teacher who radiated a living expression of health and healing. For example, one night we were sitting on the veranda of the hotel, listening to his lecture on herbs when we heard a rattlesnake. Dr. Christopher never paused for a moment as the snake crept up on the veranda and coiled up on one side of his chair. Just as we were starting to breathe easier, another snake approached and settled on the other side of Dr. Christopher. It was as if the living *Caduceus*, the curving snakes symbol of the divine physician, had manifested before our eyes. Two brothers quietly left from the back of the veranda and returned with forked stakes and nets to capture the two snakes and put them in a barrel so they could be driven out into the desert the next day. When I told Dr. Christopher that the manifestation of the snakes was an oracle in honor of his teaching, symbolizing the caduceus and the divine god of healing, *Aesclepius*, he laughed and said. "That's really wonderful."

The next afternoon when I went to see if he needed anything I saw him throwing bees out of his house from a jar. "What on earth is going on?" I asked him as I tried to enter his house.

"Be careful," he called out and I could see why. The entire house was buzzing with the biggest blackest most buzzingest bees I had ever seen. He was in the midst of them, unharmed, filling up his jar and trying to throw them out but they were coming in just as fast as he was throwing them out.

"Look, we have to plug up where they are coming in," I shouted, trying my best not to be afraid.

"O.K, you do that and I'll keep collecting them," Dr. Christopher agreed.

Soon we had the bees under control and we stopped to rest. Dr. Christopher was red from the exertion. We laughed and gasped and when we had calmed down, he asked me about myself. At the end of my story I told him how I had found my spiritual teacher and described his radiance and divine beauty that transported me beyond the mind into realms of pure spirit and absolute love. At that point tears began to flow from Dr. Christopher's eyes as he said, "I've always known there was someone like that. I always wanted to meet a teacher like that."

Over the following days Dr. Christopher and I shared a deep communion of respect and love that bonded our lives forever as teacher and student. On the last day of the seminar after all the students turned in their assignments, he again let tears flow as he returned my work to me in front of the class, with a profound look of love saying, "Without a doubt, this is the finest chart that has ever been handed in to me in all my years of teaching."

Needless to say, I was very moved. Later he came over to me and said, "This work is your destiny. You have done this in other lifetimes." When I tried to protest, he quieted me, held my hand, looked into my eyes and said simply, "Trust me. The way will open. This is your destiny."

His praise honored the vision that allowed me to see the iris chart in a new way in my mind's eye. I had drawn it on my chart as if it were a hologram, showing how the iris depicted the whole body, mind and spirit, depicting the spiritual flame coming into the crown chakra and the pranic interplay into the higher brain centers. I also showed visually how the digestive tract influences every part of the body. Iridology seemed a living part of me, as natural as breathing. I sensed and felt connections and information that Dr. Christopher hadn't even mentioned. It was as if I knew it from the inside out.

I purchased a copy of his new book, *School of Natural Healing*, and after he left I began to study regularly everyday. The week after he left I made him a large cardboard poster of my own reflexology chart that he had admired during his visit and sent it to him. A few days later he called me on the phone to thank me. I wrote him letters from time to time to tell him how my work and studies were progressing.

After his departure deep autumn glowed golden, and the community focus turned to the land and the harvest. The days were hot and sunny. Life was good. However, as the months turned from fall to winter, the leaders became stricter. Old members left and new ones arrived, with different ideas, and I began to feel uncomfortable with the excessive asceticism and the attitude that practically everything that was food was poison. I tried to remain neutral and concentrated on my spiritual path, rising at 3 a.m. to meditate, so that I could do personal creative work until 6 a.m., and then devote myself to the community and karma yoga until the afternoon rest period. I went to bed early and kept to myself, feeling that a change was coming, but not knowing what, and how or where I would go. It was too late to return to Palm Springs, so I waited for a new door to open.

The change came as a Christmas eve surprise when a satsangi on the same spiritual path telephoned, saying that he was visiting from England and wanted to come by that evening. I was happy to hear from a satsangi so I responded, "Sure, come join us for Christmas." I picked him up at the bus stop about midnight and we sat by the fire in the common room to get acquainted. A mutual friend had told him where I was and suggested that he should visit after his trip to the Grand Canyon and the Painted Desert.

The next day I realized he had more serious intentions when he began to talk about marriage, confiding that he had purposely come here to see if I was someone he would like to marry. We seemed to get along and he seemed like a fine person, so I agreed to visit him in England with the children. When he proposed, confiding honestly that he wanted to marry someone like myself, I felt it was God's will. The change had come.

Medicine Woman

The children and I moved to Cambridge, England, and I married in March. My practice and teaching started quite naturally. Nearly every person I met wanted to be either a patient or a student when they heard about my involvement with natural healing. The change was not easy. Country, culture, climate, marriage, setting up a new home – all was new and challenging. My sense of destiny supported me through the transition and meditation helped to keep me in balance and make daily life smooth. I had a clear sense that, difficult as it was for me in a new country, this was what I was supposed to do. I transformed my homesickness for my America, the desert, the free lifestyle, into an increasing passion for teaching and writing. I became a pioneer of natural healing in England, and soon I realized Dr. Christopher's words had come true, "Now

that you know the truth of this work from your own experience and my teaching, read a thousand eyes and treat those people. Then you will really know this work."

And that is exactly what I did as the years passed. My need to give and receive love became channeled into a caring profession, and I was deeply immersed in the creative process, enjoying developing the work in England. The seminars developed into a School of Natural Medicine. My practice flourished both in Cambridge and in London in Harley Street and South Kensington. I worked with medical doctors and gynecologists, receiving referrals. Medical tests taken before and after my treatment confirmed positive results. My herbal pharmacy grew into a large herb company called *Herbs of Grace*. This was also the name I gave to the guide I wrote for students and clients, which is now this book, *Herbs of Grace*. I authored two correspondence courses in Iridology and Herbal Medicine, which students subscribed to from all over the world. My husband and I co–authored both *Science and Harmony of Nature* and *Natural Fertility Awareness*. I also wrote *Iridology – a complete guide to diagnosing through the iris and to related forms of treatment*, a hardback textbook published by the Thorsons division of HarperCollins.

During this period I took fifteen trips to India to sit at the feet of my spiritual teacher. Three of the trips also included purification treatments at the Institute of Naturopathic and Yogic Sciences in Bangalore. Seven times I explored Greece, visiting different islands and areas, paying homage to ancient oracular sites such as Delphi and Eleusis, healing aesclepions like Epidaurus, and the homes of the Gods at Mt. Olympus. Over the years Crete, Rhodes, Kythera, Lesbos, Hydra and mainland Greece seemed more home to me than England. The mythic atmosphere, the colors of the sky and sea, the magic potential of ancient history, the colorful relaxed friendliness of the Greeks and their intangible mysteries nourished and healed the many conflicts and stresses of my busy life in England.

My travelling had begun in 1979 when I made my first trip to my spiritual ashram in India, Dera near Beas in the Punjab. During my month and one–half stay I worked with many Indian patients and after helping one woman who had sores all over her feet, I accidentally touched my mouth during my search for the antiseptic to wash my hands. I knew I was infected and by the next morning my body was processing the poison. As the infection worked its way through my healthy immune system I drank only water or my own urine and avoided all food for five days. When the staff heard of my illness the doctor visited me and insisted on giving me antibiotics. Before taking them I had done quite well, but the antibiotics created toxicity and liver damage, which could be seen in my iris as darkness in the liver and lymphatic zones.

When the medication finally surfaced during a healing crisis two years later, my youngest daughter, Chalice, helped me through my healing. Each morning I felt weak from toxins. After pouring an Epsom salts bath and preparing an enema for me, she helped me out of bed. The enema helped clear my system which returned to normal functioning after she gave me a lymph massage. I was then able to work throughout the day, but the next morning the toxicity returned, and we applied the same treatment. After seven days on this program the symptoms cleared, the darkness left my iris as it cleared out of my body, and life returned to normal. I share these healing experiences to demonstrate that when we meet health challenges with wisdom, knowledge and practical tools, we can clear the the difficulty and move on.

And move on I did. In 1981 I made a five–month trip back to America. After a short visit to the Santa Fe School of Natural Medicine, I completed a course for my Herbalist Diploma in Utah with the School of Natural Healing and Dr. Raymond Christopher. It was wonderful to see him again. When I invited him to come to England and teach a seminar in November he was very excited, saying that it was a dream come true, something he had always wanted to do. I was delighted that I could make a dream come true for him.

From June to October that summer and autumn of 1981, my children and I stayed at Alive Polarity centers, first on Orcas Island while we took the Basic program and then at the Napa Valley Calistoga hot spring resort, where I set up an herbal pharmacy and dispensary and put the staff on purification and rejuvenation programs. Jefferson and Sharon, the founders of the Polarity community, and I collaborated on a lymph massage technique to support purification and included it in the healing programs.

Dr. Christopher came to England in November, but later that winter he slipped, fell and was injured. A short time later passed away. I realized I was one of his disciples who would carry the torch of the teachings he had given me. It was at that time that I named my school and dedicated myself with fresh enthusiasm to sharing the healing work with patients and students.

Now that I was back in England abundance continued to manifest. My seminars, my practice and the *Herbs of Grace* herbal company blossomed. As my children were now studying and living away from home most of the time, I had more time to devote to creative work. Soon we needed five staff members to keep the office and dispensary running. However, as the outer activities increased, the inner also demanded attention. Things needed to change once more.

Personal healing during this busy time took the form of extensive deep inner explorations with the support of acupuncture, rolfing, Alexander technique, polarity therapy and cranial sacral bodywork. These therapies loosened the roots of inborn patterns, changed my posture, repositioned my spine and softened both sensory and motor receptivity and action, preparing me to delve even deeper into my interior being.

From my fortieth to forty–fifth years I plunged deeply into the shadow self, facing the darkness within until my consciousness accepted the humanity of each of the chakras, my repressions, denials, weaknesses and failures. I discovered Carl Jung and transformed what he described as shadow energies into the light, integrating them into my being and changing my personality as the individuation process matured. I changed from a martyr personality unable to ask for what I wanted or express any anger to a clear, strong, person that began to take charge of my life and find a new, realistic and direct way of being. This process, painful, exciting, mysterious and dramatic, altered all my previous patterns and moved me eventually from Cambridge back to America, but before that move could take place many significant realizations and experiences still needed to take place.

One day in London, when I saw a book in the Silver Moon Bookstore on Shaftesbury Avenue, I recognized myself in the figure on the cover of *Return to the Goddes* by Pereira. My descent into the shadow self and reconnection with deep feeling and the primal ground had changed the shape of my body. Although most of my excess weight disappeared over the next three years, my body remained fuller than before. I grew to love this mature ripe woman shape.

Toward the end of this deepening process, in 1986, I experienced six weeks of depression, something which was completely new to me as my personality had always risen above difficulties through spirituality and creativity. The depth of sadness, flatness, apathy and negativity was appalling. Life seemed completely hopeless when I realized how imprisoned I was by the chains I had created around me. I sought for a way to break free of this depression but nothing worked. One morning I awoke and knew I had to go to Greece, to Delphi, to the place where ancient priestesses gave oracles to seekers. Within a week my school secretary, Sue, and I were driving to over the mountains to Delphi, through the May countryside, fragrant and blooming with golden yellow Broom and wildflowers. That night, on the eve of my forty–fourth birthday, after visiting the oracular pools and climbing the smooth worn steps into the ancient centre of the world, I was given a visionary dream.

First I experienced myself standing with my hands above my head and behind my back. My hands were moving very, very, very slowly, endlessly, through infinite time and space toward something I could not see. As my arms finally reached the top of my head I saw a magnificent broad sword in my hands and felt tremendous weight as this sword slowly, ever so slowly, descended down, the blade glittering and shining as it caught the light in its jewels and carvings. Then before me I saw a writhing ball of threads, a huge knot. Every string represented attachments, connections, karmas, all woven together symbolizing my English destiny – husband, children, home, neighbors, friends and hundreds of patients and students. Then the sword moved with a flash and descended cleanly, clearly, to cut through the knot. The strings of light flew apart, creating an explosion that woke me up. I sat in the darkness the rest of the night, shaking and excited, as I remembered the beauty and truth of the dream.

The next morning I awoke in the best of spirits. My depression was gone and I knew what I had to do. My Gordian knot had been cut, and I was free to move on. When I returned from Greece I told my husband I would be leaving him and going back to America, and over the next few months that truth became my next reality. As an intermediary step while karmas and destinies sorted themselves out, I moved my school and *Herbs of Grace* from our large home outside Cambridge to a 16th century inn called *Dolphin House*, on Gold Street in Saffron Walden, Essex.

Although it was my deepest wish to separate from my marriage peacefully and remain friends, it was not to be. He chose to act out his anger and grief instead of taking internal responsibility for his own feelings. Instead of the divorce proceedings being a respectful mediation and clearing they became the ground for dispute. When I went to India in March of 1987 to visit my spiritual teacher I also took a rejuvenation program at the Institute of Naturopathic and Yogic Sciences in Bangalore. When I returned home my husband had moved my and my children's personal possessions out of our house into my school. His legal council advised me that I could not go back into my home.

This betrayal was a deep shock to me, and against everything we had mutually agreed upon. I plunged deeply into grief, waking up sobbing, bursting into tears several times a day and going to sleep sobbing. It was as though every wound and every sadness had collected in one place through this deep betrayal. By the time this grieving dissolved at the end of three weeks I had developed acute pain in my knees. I couldn't walk properly and was no longer able to sit on my knees or cross legged. However, so many things needed to be done that I lived with the symptoms, thinking they would go away.

When the pain did not subside I booked three weeks in December at the Institute of Naturopathic and Yogic Sciences in Bangalore and underwent the deepest purification since I had healed my breast cancer. During my consultation they examined my knees, took X–rays and advised me I had arthritis. I began a lemon water fast, which was supported by water therapies, herbal enemas, massages, steams, saunas, physiotherapy, mud treatments, yoga, pranayam, exercise and color therapy sunbaths. On the eleventh day at about five o'clock in the morning, I experienced severe diarrhea, something very rare in my life, both in daily life and during healings. Until about ten o'clock my bowels cramped in painful spasms and released small black pellets of fecal matter. Then I was fine for the rest of the day until the same time the next morning when the cycle repeated. I had thought my bowels were already empty after so many days of fasting and enemas, but each morning this cleansing repeated. After three days of this natural healing crisis my knees were no longer swollen and all the hard crystals I could feel in the tissues whenever I touched my knees had disappeared. All pain was gone and I could sit cross legged once again. I began to eat normally, pleased with the results that this fast had given me.

I do not like to think what life would have been like if I had not been able to clear these toxins out of my body and move on. I also did my best to practice mental forgiveness and to release the emotional wounds. Although my husband's behavior was a betrayal and a deep wound, it showed me what I had always known instinctively, that he was not my true friend. That was why I did not want to spend the rest of my life with him. It also gave me the opportunity to detach completely and begin my own life. In the end I chose to let go of my home and the financial settlements that were due me. I refused to go to court. I chose insted to accept the small settlement he was willing to provide because I knew entanglement with him over many months and perhaps years would not be good for me, physically or emotionally.

I surrendered to the will of the Lord and I was provided for. Unexpectedly a school graduate bought my herb company, and I was able to sell my Saffron Walden lease for more than I had paid for it. Then I received double my money when I transferred English pounds to American dollars. In September 1987, on a trip to attend a seminar in Colorado, I fell in love with Gold Hill, a mountain community in the foothills of the Rocky Mountains above Boulder. I bought a beautiful dome on three acres of open meadowland. In England I could not have bought anything at that price. Resettling myself and my two daughters was not easy and there were difficult times that we had to weather because I let go of what was due me from my divorce but I have never regretted my decision to leave England and move to Colorado. From the moment I moved into my new home in February 1988, my new life reflected the inner work that I had been doing for years under difficult circumstances. Now, at last, the outward circumstances became abundant and graceful, and my life flowed forward without resistance, as I began to enjoy my new home, 'Wisdome'. International trips from Colorado to Cambridge, England, continued as I completed my work there with students and patients. New branches of the school developed in Boulder, Colorado, and Kuala Lumpur, Malaysia.

I learned to live again, and to enjoy friends, outdoor hikes, skiing and creative dance. During my stays at the dome I wrote the Naturopathy course and began to update, improve and

extend all the school publications and teaching materials. A sense of adventure took over and I bought a four wheel drive Nissan Pathfinder to negotiate the precipitous mountain roads. I also gave attention to the buildings and the land – renovated the dome, deepened the well, designed a sacred geometry mandala deck that circled the dome with a medicine wheel four petal flower composed of two crossing vesica pisces, created a new circular doorway that opened up the dining area to the meadow and the rising sun, built a pentagon studio and a Japanese wood fired hot tub. My friends and I raised a sweat lodge and a tipi that we used throughout the beautiful snowy winters and during the summer school.

Healing for me at this time consisted of long rests after each return to the dome. Sometimes for as long as seven or even ten days I would do nothing but sleep, take aromatherapy baths, sunbathe, meditate, take walks and look at the beautiful views. It was the first time in my life I was alone, surrounded by nature and able to be my true self. During this time I created the dances that have developed into the Elemental Energetics workshops. These therapeutic visionary dances were part of my healing process after so many stressful years in England. They enabled me to reconnect to the elements of earth, water, fire, air and ether within and without, as well as releasing and dispersing blocked energies and emotions. The dances offer direct experience of the energy of the elements and their participation in the healing process. They have been integrated into the school programs to create an energy field for learning and growth.

In September 1989, after the first Colorado summer school where we welcomed students from the UK, Spain, Canada and from all over the USA, I went out to South Africa to teach two extended seminars to over one hundred students near Johannesberg. Before this trip the Iridology textbook was released by Thorsons publishers in the U.K. The school also completed the publication of the *Iridology Coloring Book* and the *Dictionary of Iridology* with Ghatfan Safi.

Just when everything seemed to be going well, I received another shock. The graduate to whom I had entrusted the British School of Iridology and the U.K. branch of the School of Natural Medicine closed the school without notice, cut off all my income and started his own school from the contacts he had made. Once again, the shock of betrayal entered my life, but this time I released it quickly. After sending a mailing to the students advising them of the difficulties, I agreed to support the completion of their correspondence studies from the Colorado school and continue to teach summer schools in England. I also opened an office on Pearl Street in downtown Boulder to develop the school and the practice locally.

The local efforts bore fruit and my living was again assured, but there seemed no hope of making my usual pilgrimage to India. In January of 1990 I received a telephone call from one of my students in Malaysia, inviting me to come out and teach a seminar. This allowed me to visit India, and then teach an Iridology and Natural Medicine seminar to over fifty students in Kuala Lumpur. I also negotiated the founding of a branch of the School in Kuala Lumpur. After the seminar I took a trip to Bali where I explored the mountain regions around Ubud and the ocean by Chandidasi. My trips to the far east were possible once again, with the added advantage that they were completely paid for by my teaching in Malaysia. I love the phrase, 'God works in mysterious ways,' because it is truly amazing how everything works out. Again and again I have experienced that there is no need to worry.

1990 became the year to deepen roots, assess motivation, clarify purpose, direction and goals for the future. It was the year to lay the structure to integrate all aspects of the healing process and offer a facility to give students the opportunity to focus on in–depth work. It was also the year to create new teaching methods that would create a group atmosphere of receptivity and awareness, to focus more on developing the internal healer within each student and to build the summer school around an in–depth study of the elements of life which has formed the ideological basis for every system of medicine in history in every part of the world, except for modern medicine.

Another shock came in June, 1990, when I received news that my spiritual master had passed on. I experienced deep grief combined with apathy. When my students arrived for the summer school I told them about my grief and asked for their support and understanding. This established an atmosphere of honesty, closeness and sharing that created a very special memory for the students who had come from the U.K., Israel, the Caribbean, the United States and Canada. However, after the students departed, the apathy, grief and fatigue did not, so I went to the island of Kauai, Hawaii. Even though I decided to go less than a week before departure, tickets were available on the fourth of July, and friends on Kauai had a room available on that day, for the exact length of my stay.

Although I had imagined that I would lie on the beach like a psychological invalid, by the second day all my grief had vanished and I was swimming and playing in the warm waters and walking on the beaches. The magical love of Hawaii embraced me once again and the sea healed my grief. When I remembered that the homeopathic remedy, Nat Mur, was the remedy for grief, divine synchronicity seemed like divine humor. Once again I had received what I needed when I needed it most, and in a most wonderful way. Although intense and excessive emotions may seem justified by great loss or shock, their effect on body, mind and spirit cannot be underestimated. I had learned again and again the effect of emotions on the physical, and longed for the spiritual grace to be able to feel deeply but have the strength to release before indulgence caused illness or imbalance.

Once again in the early spring of 1991 the way opened for me travel to India through my teaching in Malaysia. In July we held the Colorado Summer School, and in September after returning from my English summer school, I experienced deep exhaustion. For six weeks I could only rest, sleep, take baths and meditate, but the fatigue did not improve. Then one morning my instinct told me that it was time to take a break from my busy life. I had no energy to do anything so I might as well have an extended healing vacation.

Once again, everything fell into place and in one week I rented my house for six months and left the school in the capable hands of my oldest daughter, Casel. After two therapeutic weeks on the tropical Hawaiian island, Kauai, and a week in Malaysia promoting the school, I travelled to India to attend spiritual satsangs in Delhi and Bombay with the new teacher who had been appointed by my guru. After a visit to the Ajanta and Ellora caves, magnificent 9th to 13th century cave temples carved from solid rock, one of the world's greatest wonders, I went to the Institute of Naturopathic and Yogic Sciences in Bangalore for a month. During this visit I fasted eighteen days and emerged clean, clear and light and wonderfully rested.

After I left the Institute I stayed for three weeks at Kovalum Beach near Trivundrum in Kerala at the southernmost tip of India. This proved a playful celebration after such a deep purification, and I enjoyed swimming and walking on the shores of the Indian ocean. This play was followed by a visit to friends in Jaipur, Rajasthan and in Mussoorie in the foothills of the Himalayas. One month at my ashram in the Punjab was completed by another Delhi satsang. On the way home I visited Kuala Lumpur to give two seminars. I then went on to crown the trip with another two weeks on Kauai in Hawaii. Years of service, creativity and responsibility had taken their toll. Letting go and taking the time to rest, heal, have a holiday and rejuvenate had given me a new beginning. When I returned to Colorado I realized I needed to simplify, clear and reorganize my life. I knew a new creative cycle was coming and it was time to prepare. The next task was to streamline and simplify my life.

During 1994, at the age of 52, I am still experiencing the challenges and creativity of menopause. Consciously working with the energies of transformation I am moving into a new phase of my life. If any of the typical menopausal symptoms appear, whether they are hot flashes, irregular cycles, emotions or confusion, I work with them, seek to understand their purpose and what my body, mind and spirit need to do and clear the symptoms. This is a very exciting time for me, the happiest time of my life. Enjoying the fruits of my labors is complemented by the great freedom and creativity that still lies ahead.

For me menopause is a movement upwards. It is a time to release everything that moves downward and outward and of every uncompleted or resistant energy. I am enjoying awakening every part of my life and being with clarity, light and order. I am now the child within the wise woman. The happiness that accompanies the simplicity of daily life is a great gift.

This simplicity suits me well. Now I combine intense creative cycles in Boulder with healing journeys and international teaching. At the end of August 1993, after completing the Summer School, I was ready, once again, to travel. I visited Big Island in Hawaii, gave an Elemental Energetics seminar on Kauai, a menopause lecture and a workshop in Perth, Australia, and in Kuala Lumpur, Malaysia. My agenda this winter of 1994 includes writing projects and further developments in the school teaching programs. Teaching trips to Santa Barbara and Vancouver, British Columbia, support the growing work of my daughter Casel and my sister Thais, as they manifest their life journeys as medicine women. I look forward to adding more to my life story as it unfolds, and to sharing with my clients, students and readers the deepest purpose of my life and work.

I once asked Dr. Christopher what he thought the deepest purpose of his work was. After some reflection, he said very clearly, "We prepare people for better things to come." I have always held his words at the heart of my work because in my own healing I have experienced how purification creates space, how regeneration creates a new body in that space and a higher vibration to serve as a vehicle for love and truth, and how transformation is an on–going process that uplifts us for our highest purpose of receptivity to the spiritual life and its reflection in our daily life. I thank the Creator for this opportunity for service and I welcome all students and clients who seek this truth to manifest in their lives. We are all very blessed to have this work as a part of our lives.

Remember, healing is a continuum. Healing your life is a constant daily process that requires great flexibility as new doorways open after the closing of the old. I can look at my life and see the sacrifices and changes that I made in my search for truth, love, wisdom and light and see what could be called instability or mutability, but the results of the risks speak for themselves, as well as continuous joyful creativity, success, a free and wonderful daily life, loving relationships with students, clients and friends all around the world, daily work that is rewarding, continuous evolution, and flexibility to travel, explore, heal and enjoy solitude. My life feels very rich in the ways that are important to me. I focus on developing my own life because I know that what I share in my work is what I am. The quality of what I share is important to me and is my first priority. I am continuously creative in ways that reduce overhead and administration costs so that time, money and energy can lovingly be used for the most important work of service.

Each year of our lives we have the opportunity to unfold into a fuller aspect of ourselves. If we pay attention to this exquisite unfolding growing edge that is striving to be born, we do not get drawn into the negativity or fear associated with the parts of oneself that are dying away. This unfolding center is given space to grow within our being if we can let go of what no longer serves our purpose. We are constantly dying and being reborn. Conscious acknowledgment of our phoenix nature helps hold our attention in the present to make the most of the creative opportunity for growth, evolution and personal fulfillment.

The *Herbs of Grace* natural herbs, diet and therapies provide the space through purification and nutrient to regenerate and raise the body's vibratory level. As positivity gains ascendancy over negativity we automatically attain our next level of evolution. When the physical body changes, emotional and mental changes follow. As the emotions change, so does the physical and mental. As the mental attitudes change, so do the emotions and the physical body. We approach healing from all three perspectives at the same time. All the principles we use are true for each aspect, physical, emotional and mental. As the microcosm seeks alignment and harmonious resonance with the macrocosm by attuning to divine laws and putting them into practice in daily life, our healing manifests every year of our lives until we look back, as I do now, and wonder at the magic journey of my life as it moves towards the light.

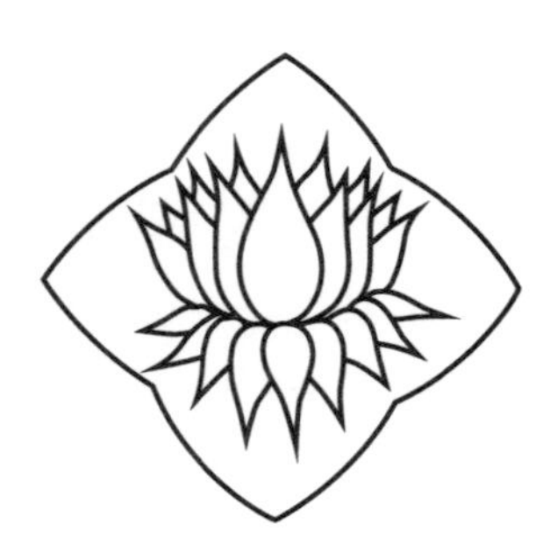

Alkaline Foods (80% of diet)

Fruits
Apples
Apricots
Avocados
Bananas (ripe)
Berries (all)
Cantaloupe
Carob, pod only
Cherries
Currants
Dates
Figs
Grapes
Mangoes
Melons (all)
Olives (fresh)
Papayas
Peaches
Pears
Raisins

LEMONS & LIMES
Citrus fruits are acidic, yet because of their high calcium content they produce an alkaline effect during the digestive process. People can experience citrus fruits as acid or as alkaline.

Vegetables
Asparagus, ripe
Aubergine
Beans –
green,
lima, string,
sprouts
Beets and tops
Broccoli
Cabbage (red & white)
Carrots
Celery
Cauliflower
Chard
Chicory
Chives
Cowslip
Cucumber
Dandelion greens
Dill
Dock, green
Dulse, seaweed
Endive
Garlic
Kale
Lettuces
Mushrooms (most)
Parsnips
Peppers (green & red)
Potatoes (all)
Pumpkin
Radish
Swede
Sorrel
Soybeans
Spinach
Spring greens
Squash
Turnips and tops
Watercress

Dairy Products
Acidophilus
Buttermilk
Milk (raw)
Whey
Goats milk yogurt

Flesh Foods
None

Cereals
Millet
Corn, green (first 24 hours)

Miscellaneous
Agar–agar
Alfalfa products
Apple cider vinegar
Coffee substitutes
Ginger, dried
Honey
Kelp
Tisanes or herb teas –
mint
clover
alfalfa
mate, sage

Nuts
Almonds

Alkalizers
Cold showers
Love
Laughter
Hugs
Fresh air

Acid Foods (20% of diet)

Fruits
Citrus fruits
Chestnuts (roasted)
Coconuts (fresh)
All preserves,
  jellies and jams
  canned
  sugared
  glazed
  fruit
Bananas, green
Cranberries
Plums
Prunes and prune juice
Olives and all pickles

Vegetables
Asparagus tips
Beans (all)
Brussel sprouts
Chickpeas
Lentils
Onions
Peanuts
Rhubarb
Tomatoes

Dairy Products
Butter
Cheese (all)
Cottage cheese
Cream, ice cream
Custard
Milk (boiled, cooked,
  dried, pasteurized,
  canned)

Flesh Foods
All meat and fowl
All fish, shellfish
Gelatin
Gravies

Cereals
All flour products
Buckwheat
Barley
Breads, all kinds
Cakes
Corn, cornmeal,
  flakes
Crackers, all biscuits
Doughnuts
Dumplings
Macaroni, spaghetti
Noodles
Oatmeal
Pies and pastry
Rice
Rye-Crisp

Nuts
All nuts (more so if
  roasted)
Coconut,
  dried
Peanuts

Neutral
Oils: olive, corn
  cottonseed, soy,
  sesame, etc.
Fat

Miscellaneous
Alcohol
Candy
Cocoa
Chocolate
Coca–Cola
Coffee
Condiments
Dressings
Sauces
Drugs (aspirin etc.)
Eggs (esp. the whites)
Ginger, preserve
Jams, Jellies
Flavorings
Marmalades
Preservatives
Corn flour
Soda water
Tobacco
Vinegars – rice, wine, etc.

Acidifiers
Lack of sleep
Overwork
Worry
Tension
Anger
Jealousy
Resentment

Acidity Remedies
Lemon juice with
  1 tsp. cider vinegar;
  add hot water and
  honey
Calcium
Nat. Phos. tissue salt

High Sources of Nutrition in Herbs and Food

	Herbs	Foods
Bromine	Bladderwrack	watermelons, celery, other melons
Calcium	Comfrey, Horsetail, Oat straw, Marshmallow, Licorice, Red Clover, Hawthorn berries	sesame seeds, seaweeds, kale, turnip, almonds, soybeans
Chlorine	Kelp	tomato, celery, lettuce, spinach, cabbage, kale, parsnip
Copper	Ephaedra	peach, turnip
Iodine	Black Walnut, Irish Moss, Kelp, Iceland Moss, Bladderwrack	turnip, dulse, seaweed
Iron	Red Raspberry, Yellow Dock, Kelp, Dandelion, Gentian	dulse, wheat and rice bran, wheat germ, pumpkin, squash and sesame seeds
Manganese	Comfrey, Cramp bark, Uva Ursi, Gravel root, Oat straw	apples, peaches, rye, turnips
Magnesium	Valerian, Kelp, Dandelion	wheat bran and germ, almonds, cashews
Potassium	Kelp, Dulse, Irish Moss, Cayenne	soybeans, bananas, beans, peas
Silica	Marestail, Oat straw	lettuce, parsnips, asparagus, dandelion greens
Sodium	Marigold, Bladderwrack, Cayenne Irish Moss, Kelp	olives, seaweeds
Sulphur	Kelp, Black Cohosh, Dandelion	onion, watercress, garlic
Phosphorus	Kelp	rice & wheat bran, wheat germ, pumpkin, squash, sesame and sunflower seeds, sesame seeds, brazil nuts
Zinc	Red Raspberry, Eyebright, Alfalfa, Uva Ursi, Slippery Elm, Hydrangea, Cramp bark, Echinacea, Yellow Dock	apricots, peaches
Vitamin A	Alfalfa, Oat straw, Cayenne, Ginger	carrots, mustard greens, asparagus, dandelion greens, docks, sorrel, kale, spinach, cress, sweet potatoes, parsley, apples, garlic, papayas, rye

High Sources of Nutrition in Herbs and Food

	Herbs	Foods
Vitamin B1 – Thiamine	Oat straw, Red Clover, Alfalfa Ginger	rice bran, wheat germ, sunflower seeds, sesame seeds, apples, garlic, papayas, turnips, rye
Vitamin B2 – Riboflavin	Alfalfa, Oat straw, Red Clover Ginger	hot red peppers, almonds, wheat germ, millet, apples, garlic, rye
Vitamin B3	Alfalfa, Red Clover, Ginger	apples, garlic, onions, papayas, parsley, rye, turnips, watercress, wheat
Vitamin B5 – Pantothenic Acid	Barberry	rye, turnips, garlic, papayas, parsley
Choline	Dandelion	parsley, turnips
B12	Alfalfa, Comfrey, Red Clover	rye, sprouted seeds, legumes
B17	Comfrey, Cramp bark, Uva Ursi, Gravel root, Oat straw	apricots, peach seeds
Vitamin C	Alfalfa, Barberry, Hawthorn berries, Marigold, Rosehips	oranges, apples, watercress, garlic, sweet red peppers, onions, turnips, black currants, parsley, walnuts, lemons
Vitamin D	Alfalfa, Fenugreek	apples, watercress
Vitamin E	Alfalfa, Flaxseed, Marigold, Rosehips, Peppermint	apples, parsley, rye, wheatgerm oil, watercress, wheat, soybean oil
Vitamin F & FF	Red Clover, Evening Primrose, Borage	garlic
Vitamin K	Alfalfa, Oat straw	apricots, garlic
Vitamin P – Rutin	Oat straw	buckwheat
Niacin	Kelp	rice & wheat bran, hot dry pepper, wild rice, sesame & sunflower seeds
Protein	Spirulina	almonds, pumpkin & squash seeds, wheat germ, dulse, beans, lentils, peas, sunflower seeds, soybean curd (tofu), avocados, millet, brewer's yeast

The highest alkaline foods are cantaloupe, avocados, melons, chinese cabbages, olives, black currants, lettuce, watercress, chicory and carrots.

Brewer's yeast and other yeast cultures contain B vitamins, as do sprouts, Spirulina and molasses.

GLOSSARY OF IRIDOLOGY TERMS

ARCUS SENILIS – cerebral anemia displayed at the top of both irides as an opaque white covering over the top of the iris ciliary margin is the result of diminishing circulation.

AUTONOMIC NERVE WREATH – a raised circular fiber which contains the digestive zone of the iris and which relates to the functions of the autonomic nervous system.

BOWEL POCKETS – the bowel forms pockets due to gas pressure and impacted feces.

CILIARY RING – the outermost ring of the iris where the iris meets the white sclera.

COLLARETTE – another term for the autonomic nerve wreath.

CRYPTS – tiny rhombic black marks which open up on the autonomic nerve wreath.

HETERACHROMIA – a sector or zone of the iris which displays a solid color that is different than the normal iris color; not to be confused with pigmentation markings.

IRIS FIBERS – under magnification the iris reveals the individual iris fibers which radiate out from the autonomic nervous system toward the ciliary edge of the iris.

LACUNAE – structural fiber openings which expand creativity, expression and release from the emotional life; potential for toxic accumulation in the physical.

LATERAL – the outer part of the body, as in the temples of the head.

LYMPHATIC TOPHI – cloud like white shapes in the lymphatic zone of the ciliary edge reveal a lymphatic constitution or congestion; may be colored gray, white, orange or even brown as the toxic levels increase in the iris and the body.

MEDIAL – the inner part of the body, as in the nose area of the head.

MIASM – from the Greek for "defilement"; inherited ancestral disease

PUPILLARY MARGIN – the small ring immediately around the pupil; often appears granulated; often colored black, brown, rust or dark orange colors

SCLERA – the white area of the eye surrounding the iris.

SCURF RING – a dark gray, brown or black ring around the ciliary edge depicting the accumulation of toxins and insufficient function of the skin and capilliary circulation.

SENSITIVITY RINGS – circular rings, one to three deep; they stop and start in different areas; they are indicative of sensitive nervous constitutions and irritated or painful areas.

RADII SOLERIS – a constitutional line or groove that radiates out from the stomach, bowel or autonomic nerve wreath; it may stop inside the collarette, break through, or continue outward to terminate in a body, organ or gland area of the iris; it influences the function of that area and may be a funnel for toxic dispersion from the bowels through the blood and lymph.

REFLEXIVE FIBERS – swollen raised thick iris fibers; can be pale pink, pink or even intensely red; indicative of inflammatory, irritated and painful conditions.

Index

A

Abdominal Packs, **96**, 99, 153
Acid/Alkaline balance, 91
Acid foods, list of, 207
Acidity remedies, 207
Acupuncture, 64, 129, 147, 159
  for cravings, 87
  for prolapse, 128
Addictions, 55, 83
Adrenal formula, 41, **52**, 62, 77, 97, 147, 155, 159
Adrenal system, 69, 72
Air element, 14, 24, 25, **32–33**
Alcohol, 84, 207
Alexander technique, 129–30
Alfalfa, 59, 64, 72, 73, **85**, 208, 209
Algaes, 155
Alive Polarity center, 116, 198
Alkaline diet, 86
  for Anxiety Gastric type, 159
  for Circulatory Hardening type, 157
  for Mixed Color type, 161
  for Velvet Brown type, 163
Alkaline foods, list of, 206
Alkaline formula, **53**, 55, 56, 73, 77, 86, 151, 159, 163
Allergies, 52
Allergy formula, **53**, 99
Allspice, 45, 74
Almond milk, how to make, 85
Almond oil, 101, 188
Aloe Vera, 97, 124, 189
  for herpes, 121
Anahata chakra, 32
Anemia formula, **53**, 73, 74, 78, 155, 161, 163
Angelica, 69
Aniseed, 54, 62, 72, 92
Anorexia, 55
Antibiotics Naturally formula, **54**, 56 63, 72, 77, 103, 120, 145
Anti–Inflammatory formula, **55**, 56, 151
Antispasmodic tincture, 47
Anti–Weight and Water formula,**55**
Anxiety Gastric type, 158–59
Apis (homeopathic), 99
Arcus senilis, 210
Arnica (homeopathic), 97
Aromatherapy
  baths, 44, 89, 97, 100
  oil, 44, 102
Arsenicum (homeopathic), 99
Arthritis, 41
  formulae for, 53, 55, 56
  herbs for, 60
  sprays for, 102
Arthritis formula, **56**
Aspirin, 55, 119
Asthma, 47, 56, 75
Asthma formula, **56**, 75
Astringent enema, 108
Autonomic nerve wreath, 210
Ayurveda philosophy, 41

B

Bach, Edward, 112
Bach flower remedies, 17, 62, 64, 71, **112**, 117, 118, 159
  diets and, 88, 90
  Rescue Remedy, 97, **98**, 99, 114
  study of, 193
  taking, 113
Back to Eden (health food store), 176
Back to Eden (Kloss), 9, 60, 180, 131, 188
Balance, 14, 87, 137
Balm of Gilead ointment, 46, 21, 127
Barberry, 53, 62, 71, 209
Baths, 9, 44, 47, **100–103**
  for acute illness, 97, 98
  fasting and, 86
  for herpes, 121
  for inflammation, 99
  skin care and, 131
  for treatment discomforts, 119
Bayberry, 61, 62, 69, 73
  as enema, 72, 108
Bearberry, 121
Bee pollen, 121
Beverages, harmful, 84
Bistort, 69
Black Cohosh, 47, 55, 56, 68, 74, 208
Black Pepper, 53, 72
Black root, 66, 71
Black Walnut, 208
Bladderwrack, 53, 55, 77, 208
Blood cleansing, 46, 56, 58, 61
Blood pressure, formulae for, 62, 67
Blood Purifier formula, **56**, 149, 157, 161, 163
  for herpes, 120
Blue Cohosh, 65, 74, 78
Blue Flag, 61, 75
Blue Vervain, 47
Body Building formula, **57**, 153, 155
  poultice of, 124, 125
  for prolapse, 128
Borage, 52, 209
Boulder (Colorado), 200
Bowel cleansing, 54, 58, 63, 70, 97

with alfalfa, 85
with castor oil packs, 105
with enemas, 106–10
herbs for, 60
for kidneys and bladder, 122
with *Psyllium*, 75
to reduce cravings, 83, 86
See also Enemas
Bowel pockets, 210
Bowel Rejuvenator formula, **58**, 59, 62, 69, 75, 89, 153, 155, 159, 161, 163
dosage for, 42
for herpes, 120
Bowel Vitalizer formula, 42, **59**, 62, 69, 155
Breast cancer
diagnosis of, 179
treatments for, 180, 181–82
Breast problems
poultice for, 125
tincture for, 48
Breathing, 93
Brewer, Judith, 174
Bristol Cancer Clinic (England), 20
British School of Iridology, 68, 201
Bromine, sources of, 208
Bronchitis. formulae for, 69, 75
Broom, 67, 77
Bruises
oil for, 47
remedies for, 97
Buchu, 46, 70
Buckwheat tea, 157
Buddhism, practice of, 174–76
Buddhist Zendo, 171
Bugleweed, 67, 77
Bulemia, 55
Burdock, 54, **59**, 64, 70, 71
douche, 133
enema, 108, 109
root, 53, 55, 75
seeds, 75
Burlap iris fiber structure, 138, 141, 154
Burn and Wound paste, 97, 103
Burns
formula for, 69
poultice for, 124, 125
remedies for, 97
Buscaglia, Leo, 176
Butter tablets, 40

C

Caffeine, 64
addiction to, 83
iron and, 53
Calamus, **59**, 66, 76
Calcium, 46, 72, 74, 76
sources of, 208
Calcium formula, **59**, 73, 97, 147, 153, 155, 163
California flower remedies, 113
Calistoga hot springs, 198
Calumba, 64
Cambridge (England), living in, 196–97
Cancer, 64
coffee enemas and, 109
formula for, 61
herbs for, 60
See also Breast cancer
Candida Albicans, 133
treatment for, 103–4
Cantharis (homeopathic), 97
Canyon Golf and Racquet Resort, 193
Capsicum (Christopher), 60
Capsicum, 101. See also *Cayenne*
Capsuling, 39, 40
Carmel, art gallery in, 169
Carob, 43, 77
Cascara Sagrada, 58
Castenada, Carlos, 187
Castor oil poultice, 67, 103, 125
Castor oil pack, 58, 68, 69, **105**, 147, 153, 155, 159, 161, 163
for constipation, 97, 107
for gall stones, 117, 122
in liver cleanse, 92
in prostate ovule treatment, 132
Catnip, 42, 45, 47, 71, 73
bath, 101
enema, 69, 108
tea, 69, 101
Cayenne, 53, 54, **60**, 61, 62, 66, 71, 75, 85, 208
bath, 125
heart attack, treatment for, 98
hemorrhage, treatment for, 99
in mono diet, 90
poultice, 125
powder, 98
in purification diet, 88
sensitivity to, 51, 52
stroke, treatment for, 98
in tincture, 47
Cereals
acid, 207
alkaline, 206
Cetraria, 64
Chakras, 25, 87, 187
Chamomile
bath, 64, 101
enema, 108
oil, 100
tea, 78
Chaparral, 54, **60**, 67, 71
bath, 47, 60
Chasteberry, 68
Chicken pox, 188
Chickweed, 46, **61**, 72, 78, 127
bath, 47, 61
douche, 104
in fomentations, 115
for itching, 99, 188
ointment, 46, 121
poultice, 125
Children
herbs for, 42–43
tincture for colic, 47
Chinchona (homeopathic), 98
Chiropractic, 69, 130, 155
Chlorine, sources of, 208
Chlorophyll, 108

Choline, 209
Chondrus Crispus, 64
Christopher, Raymond, 60, 105, 194–96, 198, 203
Chronic Purifier formula, **61**, 71, 120, 145, 149, 151
Ciliary ring, 210
Cinnamon, 45, 53, 54, 58, 77, 92
Circulation Cerebral formula, **61**, 67, 149, 157
Circulation Systemic formula, 61, **62**, 67, 149, 155, 157, 161
Circulatory Hardening type, 156–57
Circulatory formulae , 61, 62, 67
  herbs for, 60
Cleansing cycles, 119
Cleavers, 66
Clivers, 46, 70
Cloves, 54, 61, 64, 70
  in liver cleanse, 92
  oil from, for tooth pain, 99
  sensitivity to, 52
Coconut oil, 132
Coffee enema, 44, **109**
  in juice cleanse, 89
  substitute for, 64
Cold abdominal pack, 159
Colds and Flu formula, **63**
Colds and flu treatment, 63, 69, 98, 107
Colic
  herbs for, 78
  tincture for, 47, 48
Colitis formula, **62**
  dosage for, 41
Collarette, 210
Colocynthis (homeopathic), 97
Colonics, 58, 163
  and fasting, 86
  See also Bowel cleansing; Enemas
Colors, elemental, 24–25
  of air element, 32
  of earth element, 26
  of ether element, 34
  of fire element, 30
  of water element, 28
Coltsfoot, 76
Comfort foods, 87
Comfrey, 124, 127, 208, 209
  leaves, 57
  ointment, 46, 121, 127
  poultice, 125, 188
  for prolapse, 128
  powder, 103
  root, 53, 56, 57, 61, 67, 75, 78
Congestion
  formulae for, 76, 77
  poultice for, 48, 125
Conrad, Emily, 184
Constipation, 111
  abdominal packs and, 97
  in liver cleanse, 92
Copper, natural sources of, 208
Cotton iris fiber structure, 138, 140, 150
Couchgrass, 46
Coughing, poultice for, 48
Cramp Bark, 71, 74, 78, 208, 209
  tincture, 47
Cramps
  formulae for, 65, 78
  herbs for, 78
  remedies for, 97
  tinctures for, 47, 48
Cranial sacral, 64
Cravings, 83, 87
Crescent Beach, indian relics at, 168
Crypts, 210
Cucumber, poultice of, 124
Culver's root, 58
Cystitis, tea for, 46

D

Dairy products, 84
  as acid food, 207
  as alkaline food, 206
Dandelion, 67, 71, 72, 76, 208, 209
  coffee from, 83, 84
Death transition, 25
Decoctions, 45, 64
  of Blue Cohosh, 74
  as enemas, 108
  making, 44
  of Hydrangea, 68
  of Yellow Dock, 78
Deep tissue massage, 130, 151
Delphi (Greece), visiting, 199
Dera near Beas ashram, 197
Desert Hot Springs (California), 193
Detoxifying enema, 108
Devil's Claw, 55
Diarrhea
  dosage for, 42
  enema for, 108
  herbs for, 72
  in liver cleanse, 92
  remedies for, 98
  tea for, 46
  treatment of, 58
Dictionary of Iridology (Sharan), 201
Diets
  for Anxiety Gastric type, 159
  avoiding, 87
  for Circulatory Hardening type, 157
  effect on health, 80–81
  for Glandular Digestive type, 153
  for Immune Reactive type, 145
  for Kidney/Gall Stone cleanse, 122
  for Lymphatic Holding type, 151
  for Lymphatic Sensitive type, 149
  for Mixed Color type, 161
  Mono diet, 90
  or Nervous Sensitive type, 147
  Purification diet, 88
  for Structurally Open type, 155
  for Velvet Brown type, 163
Digestea, **45**
Digestion, 52, 69, 71, 72
  enemas for, 107
  herbs for, 59, 66, 76
  mono diet for, 90
  tea for, 45, 46

tincture for, 47
Dolphin House Inn (England), 199
Dong Quai, 72
Dosages, **41–42**
during acute crisis, 54
of Bach flower remedies, 98, 113
for children, 43
for Ear formula, 63
of Hydrangea, 68
of tinctures, 48
Douches, 66, 74, 104
equipment for, 111
of Yellow Dock, 78
Dreams, 186
Dulse, 208
Dunsmuir (California), 188
Dying persons, caring for, 43–44
Dysentery, enema for, 108

E

Earache, oil for, 47
Ear formula, **63**
Earth element, 14, 24, 25, **26–27**
Echinacea, 54, 55, 56, 61, **63**, 69, 71, 75, 78, 103, 127, 208
as douche, 104
for herpes, 120
tincture, 47
Eggs, 84
Elderflower, 55, 63, 75
tincture, 48
Elderly, dosage for, 43
Elecampagne, 53, 56, 74, 75, 124
poultice, 125
Elemental energetics, 24–35, 201
Elimination systems, 56, 58, 59, 61, 65, 67, 68
formula for, 55, 70, 71
herbs for, 66
skin disorders and, 131
Emotions, elemental, 25
of air element, 33
of earth element, 27
eating habits and, 81
of ether element, 35
of fire element, 31
of water element, 29
Enema formula, **64**
Enemas, 9, 44, 45, 54, 58, 63, 70, 72, 97, **106–10**, 163
equipment for, 111
fasting and, 86
fever and, 98
in Gall Bladder cleanse, 116
for Glandular Digestive type,153
in juice cleanse, 89
in vaginal ovule treatment, 133
Energy snacks, 91
Ephaedra, 53, 208
tea, 63
Epilepsy, tincture for, 47
Epsom salts, 100
baths of, 67, 97, 101
Esalen massage, learning, 184
Essene Gospel of Peace, The, (Szekeley), 106, 190
Estrogen, 68
Ether element, 14, 24, 25, **34–35**
Euonymous, 66
Euphrasia, tincture of, 47
Evening Primrose, 209
Exercise, 86, 93
Exhaustion, herbs for, 66
Exhaustion formula, **64**, 77, 91, 155
dosage for, 41
Extracts, from powders, 39
Eyebright, 65, 208
Eyes, tincture for, 47
Eye Wash formula, **65**

F

False Unicorn, 68
Fasting, 76, 86
purification and, 19
Spirulina enemas and, 110
Female Reproductive formula, **65**
Fennel, 42, 45, 47, 54, 70, 71
in liver cleanse, 92
seeds, 55
Fenugreek, 44, **65**, 72, 209
in liver cleanse, 92
tea, 149
Fever, 69, 98, 108
Fiber structures, of iris, 138
Fibroids, 48, 102
Fingernail ridges, 91
Fire element, 14, 24, 25, **30–31**, 83
Fish, 84, 207
Flatulence, 48, 59, 78, 108
Flaxseed, 209
enema, 108
Flesh foods, 206, 207
Flour, 84
Flower essences, 44, 55, 83, 113
Flower remedies, 98, **112–14**
making your own, 114
for prolapse, 129
Fomentations, 9, 45, 77, **115**
Food
acid food list, 207
alkaline food list, 206
beneficial, 84–86
eating habits and, 81
harmful, 84
as medicine, 81, 83
nutritional sources of, 208–9
Foot baths, 47, 102, 115
Formulae, herbal, 38–39, 50
own preparation of, 39
proportions, 51
See also Individual formulae
Fruits
acid, 207
alkaline, 206
Fungal infections, 66
Fungus/Candida formula, **66**

G

Gall Bladder cleanse, **116–18**
Gall Bladder formula, **66**
Gall stones, 117, 118
Garlic, 54, 69, 86
injection, 108
in liver cleanse, 92
oil, 47, 63

in purification diet, 88
sensitivity to, 51, 52
Gas, 106
in children, 42
from Gall Bladder cleanse, 117
herb treatment for, 78
Gentian root, 64, **66**, 70, 91, 208
Gerson, Max, 64, 109
Gerson cancer therapy programs, 20, 64, 109, 117
Gestalt group, belonging to, 184
Gibran, Kahlil, 172
Ginger, 45, 54, 56, 59, 62, 69 86, 208, 209
bath, 101, 125
in cleanses, 92, 122
for kidneys, 122, 123, 151
poultice, 68, 125, 151, 159
powder, 98
root, 53, 58, 67, 72, 78
sensitivity to, 51, 52
tea, **46**, 63
Ginseng, 52, 67, 68
sensitivity to, 52
Glandular Digestive type, 152–53
Glycerin, vegetable, 110
Goat's milk, 84, 206
Golden Door, 190
Golden Seal, 54, 58, 59, 62, 65, 69, 74, 75, 103
poultice, 125, 188
root, 78
Gold Hill, living in, 200–201
Gordian knot disease pattern, 17, 199
Gotu Kola, 52, 59, 64, **66**, 73
Gravel root, 70, 75, 208, 209
Greece, travels to, 197
Guarana, use of, 176
Guiacum, 55
Gum Myrrh, 47

H

Haiku (Maui), living in, 171–74
Hair Strengthening formula, **67**
Hakomi, 130
Haleakala, pilgrimage to, 172–73
Hand baths, 47, 102, 115
Hawthorn berries, 52, 62, 67, 208, 209
Healing
ointment for, 46
transformation and, 22
Healing Waters, 47, 194–96
Health ecology, 14–16
Heal Thyself (Bach), 112
Heart attack, treatment of, 47, 60, 98
Heart Tonic formula, **67**, 157
Heavy Metal Purifier formula, **67**, 151
Hemorrhage, 60, 99
Hemorrhoids, 128
Herbs
brewing, 41
grinding, 39
taking, 38, 52
Herbs of Grace herb company, 197
Hering's Law of Cure, 119
Herpes, 48, **120–21**
Heterachromia, 210
Hibiscus, 45
Hip baths, 102
Holy Thistle, 68, 74
Homeopathy, 44, 129
Homeostasis, 14, 20, 137
Honey, 85, 103, 125
in juice cleanse, 89
in mono diet, 90
in poultices, 126
in purification diet, 88
tablets, 40
Hook treatment, 128–29
Hops, 45, 77
Hormone Balance formula, 65, **68**, 153, 163
Hormones, 72
Hornbeam flower remedy, 64
Horsetail, 59, 72, 208
Hot Creek, bathing in, 181
Hot flashes, 48, 72
Hot Mustard bath, 54
Humors, as elements, 25
Hydrangea root, **68**, 118, 122, 208
Hyperactivity, 47, 73
Hypericum (homeopathic), 99
Hypoglycemia, 46, 74
Hypothalamus, 136

I

Iceland Moss, 53, 76, 77, 208
Ileocaecal Valve formula, **69**
Immune Reactive type, 144–45
Immune system, formula for, 53
India, travels in, 197, 202–3
Infants
calcium for, 59
herbs for, 42
Infection
enemas for, 107
formula for, 56
herbs for, 63
poultice for, 124
tincture for, 47
Infection formula, **69**, 72, 145
Inflammation
abdominal packs for, 96
enema for, 108
formulae for, 55, 56, 57
mud packs for, 97
poultice for, 48
treatment for, 99
Infusions, 44, 108, 128
Inner ecology, 14–16, 17, 50
health and, 25
Iridology and, 136–38
purification and, 18
regeneration and, 19
transformation and, 21
Inner world, 24
in health ecology, 14
nourishment and, 82
Insect bites, 99
Insomnia, 73
Institute of Naturopathic & Yogic Sciences (India), 97, 197, 199, 200, 203
Insulin, from herbs, 74

Intestinal Infection formula, **70**
Inversion therapy, for prolapse, 128
Iodine, 66, 208
Ipecacuanha (homeopathic), 98, 99
Iridology, **136–63**
  and inner ecology, 15–16
Iridology, 9, 50, 68, 74, 106, 120
  for Candida, 104
  fiber structures in, 138
  Iricology and, 136, 137
  iris constitutional types, 143–63
  in prostate ovule treatment, 132
  purification and, 18
  study of, 193, 195
Iridology – a complete guide to diagnosing through the iris and to related forms of treatment (Sharan),136, 197
Iridology Coloring Book (Sharan), 201
Iris analysis, 58, 83
  colors of, 136
  constitutional types, 143–63
  fibers in, 138, 210
  pigmentation in, 67
  See also Iridology
Irish Moss, 53, 57, 61, 73, 73, 76, 77, 208
Iron, 84
  Anemia formula for, 53
  herbs for, 78
  sources of, 208
Itching, 99, 125

J
Jamaican Dogwood, 74
Jensen, Bernard (quote by), 119
Jin jin jitsu, 130
Journey to Ixtlan (Castenada),187
Juice cleanse, 76, **89**, 122
Juice fasts, 19, 116
Juice punch, recipe for, 45
Jung, Carl, 198
Juniper
  berries, 70, 74
  oil, 100

K
Kauai (Hawaii), travel to, 202
Kava Kava, 66, 73
Kelly cancer program, 109
Kelp, 53, 59, 77, 85, 208, 209
  for herpes, 121
Kidney/Bladder formula, 67, **70**, 75, 151
  dosage for, 42
Kidney/Gall Stone cleanse, 68, 118, 122
Kidneys
  formulae for, 70, 72
  poultices for, 123, 125
  stones, 68
Kineseology, 52, 68, 69
Kloss, Jethro, 9, 60, 131, 180
Kuala Lumpur (Malaysia), 200, 201
Kwan Yin, 172

L
Lacunae, 210
Lady Slipper/Valerian formula, **71**
Lady's Slipper, 47, 64, **70**, 71, 73, 77
Lahaina (Maui), 173–74
Lateral, 210
Lavender, oil of, 100
Lecithin, 85, 88
Ledum (homeopathic), 99
Lemon
  as alkaline food, 206
  in Gall Bladder cleanse, 116
  in liver cleanse, 92
  in mono diet, 90
Lemon Balm, 78
Lemon Grass, 45
Licorice, 65, 208
  root, 53, 54, 56, 59, 68, 74, 75
  tea, **46**, 74, 92, 155
Life changes, and purification, 18
Life cycles, 10
Lightening strikes, treatment, 99
Lily of the Valley, 67
Lime, as alkaline food, 206
Lime tree, flowers of, 67, 77
Lindlahr, Henry (quote by), 119
Linen iris fiber structure, 138, 139, 146, 150
Liver Cleanse drink, 88, **92**, 157
Liver disorders, 72
Liver/Gall Bladder formula, **71**, 75, 157, 161, 163
Lobelia, 52, 53, 54, 59, 67, 69, 71, 73, 74, 75, 76, 77
  bath, 44, 47, 64, 101
  heart attack, treatment for, 98
  poultice, 76, 124, 125
  stroke, treatment for, 98
  tincture, 48
London, 193, 197
Los Angeles, art gallery in, 169
Lotus sutra, 174
Lymphatic formula, **71**, 75, 77, 99, 103, 145, 149, 151, 157
Lymphatic Holding type, 150–51
Lymphatic Sensitive type, 148–49
Lymphatic system
  formulae for, 69, 71
  herbs for, 59, 63
Lymphatic tophi, 210
Lymph massage, 109, 149
Lysine, 121

M
Macrobiotic books, 86
Magnesium, sources of, 208
Maharaj Charan Singh Ji, 193
Mammouth (California), 180
Mandalas, 185, 186, 187
Mandrake root, 59
Manganese, sources of, 208
Manipura chakra, 30
Mantra of death, 177
Marestail, 208
Marigold, 208, 209
Marshmallow, 124, 208
  poultice, 125
  root, 53, 56, 57, 59, 66, 70, 74,

75, 78
Massage, **44**, 130, 147, 155, 159, 163
and fasting, 86
Meadowsweet, 45, 66, 71, 76
Medial, 210
Medicine, elemental, 25
Meditation, 93, 159
juice cleanse and, 89
practice of, 186
Menopause, 78
experiencing, 203
formulae for, 65, 68, 72
tincture for, 48
Menopause formula, 65, **72**
Menstruation
formulae for, 65, 78
tea for, 46
Meridians, 25, 87
Miasm, 210
Milk Thistle, **72**
seeds, 75
Mimosa Gum, 61
Mineral oil, skin care and, 131
Miscarriage, 78
Miso, 83, 84, 85, 91
in purification diet, 88
Mistletoe, 45
Mixed Color type, 160–61
Modern Herbalism for Digestive Disorders (Roberts), 116
Mono diet, 19, 44, **90**
for Anxiety Gastric type, 159
for Circulatory Hardening type, 157
for Glandular Digestive type, 153
for Lymphatic Holding type,151
Morrison, Jim, 170, 174
Motherwort, 65, 67, 72
Mount San Jacinto bluegrass festival, 190
Mount Shasta, living in, 185–89
Movement classes, 184
Mucus, 56, 60
in colon, 58
juice cleanse for, 89
Mucus Congestion formula, **72**, 145
Mud packs, 97, 102
Muladhara root chakra, 26
Mullein, 52, 54, 57, 69, 70, 71, **72**, 74, 75, 76, 77, 124
infusion, 98
in liver cleanse, 92
oil, 47, 63
poultice, 99, 125
tea, **46**, 58, 72
Multi–Minerals/Vitamins Naturally formula, 41, **73**, 77, 86, 91, 103, 153, 159
Muslin iris fiber structure, 138, 140
Mustard
bath, 63, 69, 101, 125
poultice, 125
powder, 98
Myrrh, 62, 66, 70
tincture, 48, 121

N

Nam Myoho Renge Kyo, 174
Napa Valley resort, 198
Nat Mur, homeopathic grief remedy, 202
Natural childbirth, 169
Natural Fertility Awareness, 197
Natural fibers, 93
Nausea, from Gall Bladder cleanse, 117
Negative energy, 186–87
Nerve Rejuvenator formula, 41, 62, **73**, 77, 97, 147, 153, 159
for herpes, 120
Nerve rings, 210
Nerve Tonic formula, 41, 62, **73**, 77, 97, 147, 159
Nerve Vitalizer formula, 41, 62, **73**, 77, 97, 147, 159
Nervine Nutrient tincture, 47
Nervine Relaxant tincture, 47
Nervous Sensitive type, 146–47
Nervous system, 69
formulae for, 73, 77
herbs for, 66, 70
tincture for, 47
Net structure iris type, 142
Nettles, 55, 72, 74, 77
Neuromuscular massage, 130
Niacin, 209
Nichirin Shoshu, 174–76
Nicotine, 76
Nourishment, 80–82, 93
patterns of, 19–20
Nuts
acid, 207
alkaline, 206

O

Oat Straw, 59, 208, 209
tea, **46**
Oils, 47
aromatherapy, 100
in baths, 102–3
in mono diet, 90
for vaginal infections, 103
Ointments, 46
Olive flower remedy, 64
Olive oil, 67, 101
in Gall Bladder cleanse, 116
in juice cleanse, 89
as liver cleanse, 92
in purification diet, 88
Oregon Grape root, 56
Osteopathy, 69, 128, 130, 155
Osteoporosis, 48, 59
Outer ecology, and Iridology, 136–37
Outer world, 24
in health ecology, 14
nourishment and, 82
Ovule, rectal, 75

P

Pain reduction, 44
Pain Relief formula, **74**
Palm Springs, 189–90, 192–93
Pancreas formula, **74**, 161
Pannetier, Pierre, 193

Parsley, 77
  leaves, 46, 77
  in liver cleanse, 92
  root, 52, 55, 56, 59, 65, 70, 75
  tea, 122
Passion flower, 77
Pau D'Arco, tea, 97
Pendulum, 52
Peppermint, 45, 63, 71, 209
  in liver cleanse, 92
  for stomach ailments, 54
  tea, 48, 69, 98, 101
  for vomiting, 99
Phosphorous, sources of, 208
Phosphorus (homeopathic), 99
Plantain, 57, 69, 77
Pleurisy root, tea of, 101
Poke, root of, 54, 55, 56, 66, 71, 75, 125
Polarity balancing, 159
Polarity therapy, 64, 69, 92, 130, 193
Potassium, 48, 85
  sources of, 208
Potassium broth, 85, 88
Poultices, 9, 44, 45, **124–27**
  for burns, 103
  for colds and flu, 63
  from formulae, 53, 57, 66
  Ginger, 68, 123
  for infection, 63
  internal, 78
  Lobelia, 48, 76
  for prolapse, 128
  Slippery Elm, 76
  for tooth pain, 99
Poultry, 84
Powders
  alternative preparation of, 40–41
  capsuling, 40
  dosage of, 42
  drinking, 40–41
  from formulae, 65
  preparation of, 39
Pregnancy
  Anemia formula for, 53
  formulae during, 68, 74
  herbs to avoid during, 58, 59
  herb usage during, 42, 78
  tea for, 46
Pre–Natal formula, **74**
Prickly Ash, 55, 56, 61, 73
Progesterone, 48, 68, 78
Prolapse formula, **74**
Prolapse treatment, **128–29**
Prostate formula, **75**
Prostate ovule, **132–33**
Protein, 209
Prune juice, 89
Psychedelic Conspiracy boutique, 171
Psyllium, **75**
Pumpkin seeds, 70, 86
Pupillary margin, 210
Purification, 10, 17, **18–19**, 67
  acupuncture and, 129
  herbal formulae and, 50
  herbs for, 60
  as transition, 80
Purification diet, 9, 19, 44, 68, 76, **88**
  for Gall Bladder cleanse, 116
  and liver cleanse, 92
  for Lymphatic Holding type, 151
  for Velvet Brown type, 163
Pyorrhea, tincture for, 48

Q

Quassia Root, 53, 69, 70

R

Radha Soami, 193
Radii soleris, 210
Radionics, 68
Rainbow Family, living with, 190–192
Rainbow Island Healing Center, 47
Rashes, treatment for, 99
Rectal ovule, 75
Red Clover, 64, 72, 75, 208, 209
  blossoms, 56
  enemas, 108, 109
  tea, **46**, 163
Red Raspberry, 64, 65, 72, 74, 208
  enemas, 72, 108, 109
  tea, **46**, 69, 163
Referrals, to other practitioners, 129–30
Reflexive fibers, 210
Reflexology, 44, 64, 93, 130, 151, 163
  fasting and, 86
  for kidneys, 122
  in liver cleanse, 92
  for prolapse, 128
  for tooth pain, 99
  for vomiting, 99
Regeneration, 10, 17, **19–20**
  and acupuncture, 129
Reiki, 130
Rejuvenation program, 50, 67, 92
Reproductive system, formulae for, 65, 78
Rescue Remedy, 97
Respiratory disorders
  formulae for, 56, 69, 72, 75, 76
  poultice for, 125
Respiratory formula, 56, **75**
Return to the Goddess (Pereira), 198
Rheumatism
  dosage for, 41
  formulae for, 53, 55, 56
Rhus Tox (homeopathic), 99
Roberts, Frank, 116
Rolfing, 130
Rose hips, 45, 73, 209
  tea, **46**
Rosemary oil, 100
Rosen work, 130

S

Saffron, 86

Sage, 61, 67, 70
  enema, 108
  tea, **46**, 67, 101
Salt, 84
Sandalwood oil, 100
San Luis Obispo, working in, 193
Santa Fe School of Natural Medicine, 198
Santa Monica
  living in, 182–84
  studio in, 170
Santa Monica Childcare Mothers' Association, 176–77
Sarsaparilla, 53, 54, 55, 56, 68
  tea, for herpes, 120
Sassafras, 53, 54, 56
Satsangs, attending, 193, 202
Saunas, 101
  and fasting, 86
Saw Palmetto, 48, 75
School of Natural Healing, 105, 195, 198
School of Natural Medicine (England), 197, 201
Science and Harmony of Nature, 197
Sclera, 210
Scottsdale, art gallery in, 169
Scullcap, 45, 47, 67, 73, 77
Scurf ring, 210
Seaweeds, 66, 84, 86, 155
  in purification diet, 88
Sedatives, herbal, 64, 70
Sensitivity rings, 210
Sepia (homeopathic), 129
Serenitea, 45(B)
Sesame seeds, 86
Shadow self, 198
Shakamuni Buddha teachings, 174
Shakubuku, 175
Shiatsu, 64, 130
  learning, 189
Shock, 47, 73
Silica, 46
  sources of, 208
Silk iris fiber structure, 138, 139, 150
Silver Moon bookstore (London), 198
Sitz bath, 102, 121
Skin
  care of, 131
  fomentations for, 115
  formulae for, 72, 75
  herbs for, 59, 61, 65
  oil for, 47
  ointment for, 46
  tincture for, 48
Skin Problems formula, **75**
Sleep disorders
  in children, 42
  formulae for, 71
  herbs for, 70
Slippery Elm, 39, 56, 58, 62, **76**, 77, 208
  drink, 43, 52
  enema, 108
  poultices, 99, 125, 126, 127, 128
  powder, 132
  tablets, 40
  tea, 72
Smoking formula, **76**
Sodium, sources of, 208
Sore Throat syrup, 63
  recipe for, 54
Soy cheese, 84
Spearmint, tea from, 101
Spirulina, 55, 73, **76**, 84, 86, 155, 209
  bars, 91
  cravings and, 87
  enema, **110**
  in juice cleanse, 89
Sprains
  oil for, 47
  poultice for, 57, 125
Sprays, 102
Squaw Vine, 65, 68, 74, 78
St. John's Wort, 61
Steambaths, 86
Stomach Acid/Alkaline Balancing formula, 41, **76**
Stone, Randolph, 92
Strauss, Margaret, 64, 109
Stress, 64
  formulae for, 52, 73
  herbs for, 70
  herpes and, 120
  tea for, 45
Stroke
  sprays for, 102
  treatment of, 98
Structurally Open type, 154–55
Sugar, 84
Sulphur, sources of, 208
Sunburn, poultice for, 124
Sunflower seeds, 86, 87
Svadhisthana chakra, 28
Sweat lodge, 194
Sweats, 54, 63, 69
  for fever, 98
Sweet Sleep formula, 73, **77**, 147
Swelling
  formulae for, 57, 77
  oil for, 47
  poultice for, 125
  tincture for, 48
Swollen Glands formula, **77**
Syphilis, 61
Szekeley, Edmund Bordeaux, 190

T

Tableting formula, **77**
Tai chi, 93, 155, 159
Tamari, 84
Teas, herbal,
  for children, 42
  from Colds and Flu formula, 63
  for hair washing, 67
  making, 44–45
  in purification diet, 88
  types of, 45–46
  See also individual herb names
Tea Tree oil
  for vaginal infections, 103, 104

in vaginal ovule, 132, 133
Three Gong Ceremony, 184
Three–seed powder, 88
Thrush, 133
Thyme, 58, 66, 70, 103, 127
douche, 133
infusion, 126
oil, for vaginal infections, 103, 104
tea, for stomach ailments, 54
Thyroid Balancing formula, 73, **77**, 147, 153, 157, 159
Tinctures
from Blue Cohosh, 74
for children, 42–43
from Fenugreek, 65
making tea from, 44
from powders, 39
Tisanes, 44
Tofu, 84, 86
Tooth pain, treatment for, 99
Toxemia, 106
Trager work, 130
Transformation, 10, 17, **21–22**, 50
Treatise on Herbology (Shook), 53
True Unicorn, 65, 74
Tryptophan, 121
Tucson ashram, living in, 183
Turkey Rhubarb, 58
Turkish baths, 101
Turmeric, 78, 86

U
Urinary system, herbs for, 60
Uva Ursi, 46, 67, 70, 74, 208, 209
bath, for herpes, 121

V
Vaginal ovule treatment, **132–33**
Vaginal/Prostate Ovule formula, 66, 76, **78**, 104
Vaginitis, sitz baths for, 102
Valerian, 45, 70, 73, 74, 77, 78, 208
root, 71
as sedative, 64
tincture, 42, 47
tea, 42
Vancouver, living in, 168
Varicose veins, 115
Vegetables
acid, 207
alkaline, 206
Vegetarian diets, 64, 163
Velvet Brown type, 162–63
Velvet iris type, 142
Veratrum (homeopathic), 98
Vervain, 45
Vibratory affinities, and transformation, 21
Vinegar, apple cider, 85, 89
baths of, 101
for fever, 98
in mono diet, 90
in poultices, 126, 127
Violet, 72, 92
Vishudda chakra, 34
Visualization, 93, 186
Vital circuitry, 93
Vitamin A, 208
for herpes, 121
Vitamin B complex, 209
for herpes, 121
Vitamin C, 46, 209
for herpes, 120
Vitamin D, 65, 209
Vitamin E, 67, 86, 157, 209
Vitamin E oil, 103, 125
for chicken pox, 188
for herpes, 121
Vitamin F/FF, 209
Vitamin K, 209
Vitamin P (rutin), 209
Vomiting
abdominal packs for, 96
treatment of, 99

W
Wahoo, 58, 71, 74
Warner Hot Springs, 190
Warts, oil for, 47
Waterbalance tea, 46, 122
Water element, 14, 24, 25, **28–29**
Weight loss, 88, 91
Wheat germ oil, 67, 86, 103
for herpes, 121
for itching, 188
Wheatgrass juice
douche, 104
for herpes, 120
as implant, 108
poultice, 125
White Brotherhood, 171
White Oak
bark, 57, 62, 74
enema, 108
White Rock, living in, 167–68
White Willow bark, 55, 74
for tooth pain, 99
Wild Lettuce, 42, 47
Wild Yam root, 59, 71, 72, **78**
tincture, 48
Wisdome, 200
Witch Hazel, 74
enema, 72, 108
for varicose veins, 115
Women's Period Pain formula, 65, 78, **78**
Wood Betony, 45
Wormwood, 70
Wounds, poultice for, 57, 125

Y
Yarrow, 55, 67
tea, 63, 69, 98, 101
Yeast infections, 103–4
Yellow Dock, 64, 74, **78**, 208
douche, 104, 132, 133
enema, 108, 109
root, 53, 56, 67
tea, 163
Yerba Santa, 76
Yoga, 25, 93, 155, 159
Yogi Bhajan, 183

Z
Zig Zag iris fiber structure, 138, 141
Zinc, sources of, 208

School of Natural Medicine, P.O.Box 7369, Boulder CO 80306 – 7369, U.S.A.
Telephone and FAX: 303 – 443 – 4882 Director: Dr. Farida Sharan

HERBS OF GRACE – HERB ORDER FORM

The School of Natural Medicine's herbal pharmacy, Herbs of Grace, offers safe, non–toxic, non–habit forming herbal nutrient formulae created by Dr. Farida Sharan. The wildcrafted, organic, fresh ground herbal powders are blended to order, to the highest professional standard. Powders provide the purest, most easily assimilable herbal food without the addition of alcohol or the chemical changes of the extraction process. All formulae have been tried and tested by hundreds of our graduates and professionals. Complete details on all the formulae, contents and recommended use, together with information on diets and home naturopathic treatments are provided in *Herbs of Grace – Becoming Independently Healthy*, which we recommend be included with any herb order. Capsules and capsuling machines may also be ordered. Prices valid through June 1995. Please request new forms after this date.

#	Powdered Formulae per ounce	$	$ Total
	Adrenal	12.00	
	Alkaline	10.00	
	Allergy	10.00	
	Anemia	10.00	
	Antibiotic	11.00	
	Anti–Weight	12.00	
	Anti–Inflammatory	10.00	
	Arthritis	11.00	
	Asthma	11.00	
	Blood Purification	12.00	
	Body Building	10.00	
	Bowel Rejuvenator	12.00	
	Bowel Activator	12.00	
	Calcium	10.00	
	Chronic Purifier	12.00	
	Circulation Systemic	12.00	
	Circulation Cerebral	12.00	
	Colitis	12.00	
	Enema Mix	11.00	
	Exhaustion	11.00	
	Female Reproductive	12.00	
	Fungal Infection	10.00	
	Heart	12.00	
	Heavy Metal Purifier	12.00	
	Hormone Balance	12.00	
	Ileo-Caecal Valve	11.00	
	Intestinal Infection	11.00	
	Kidney/Bladder	12.00	
	Liver/Gall Bladder	12.00	
	Lymphatic	12.00	

#	Powdered Formulae per ounce	$	$Total
	Menopause	12.00	
	Multi-Mineral/Vitamins	11.00	
	Nerve Rejuvenator	12.00	
	Nerve Tonic	12.00	
	Nerve Vitalizer	12.00	
	Pancreas Sugar Balance	12.00	
	Prolapse	11.00	
	Prostate	12.00	
	Respiratory	11.00	
	Skin Clear	11.00	
	Stomach Acid/Alkaline Balance	11.00	
	Sweet Sleep	11.00	
	Thyroid	11.00	
	Vaginal Ovule +Y.D. + S.Elm	12.00	
	Women's Period Pain	12.00	
	Capsuling Machine	20.00	
	Herbs of Grace book	24.00	
	Creative Menopause book	18.00	
	Creative Menopause cassette	13.00	
	500 Gelatin Capsules	25.00	
	School Brochure	Free	

TOTAL ______

POSTAGE ______

GRAND TOTAL ______

INDICATE WHETHER YOU WANT HERBS PACKAGED SEPARATELY (S) OR BLENDED TOGETHER (B)

POSTAGE & PAYMENT INFORMATION

U.S. orders up to $50 – postage $5; orders up to $100 – postage $9.
Canadian postage airmail $9 up to $50; $13 up to $100. International orders, $20 up to $50; $30 up to $100.
Make checks payable to School of Natural Medicine
Payment in U.S. dollars, by check, m.o. or Visa /MC by phone, mail or FAX. Orders must be prepaid.

DATE .... AMOUNT IN FULL ....

NAME .... TEL. NO. ....

ADDRESS ....

.... ZIP CODE ....COUNTRY ....

VISA/MASTERCARD NUMBER .... EXPIRATION DATE ....

SIGNATURE ....

School of Natural Medicine Study Opportunities

Home Study

Correspondence home study courses in Iridology, Herbal Medicine and Naturopathy and a combined Natural Physician course are available worldwide from the Colorado branch of the international School of Natural Medicine, P.O. Box 7369, Boulder, Colorado 80306–7369. Telephone and FAX (303) 443–4882. U.S. enquirers please send $2.00, Canadians $3.00 and international students $5.00, for our extensive brochure, latest newsletter and application form.

Worldwide Seminars

A *Creative Menopause – Illuminating Women's Health & Spirituality* lecture proceeds a one or two–day workshop on *Elemental Energetics – Life in Creative Motion* or *Creative Women's Health*, original workshop processes to inspire those whose lives are in transition, who seek healing and evolution of consciousness, and who wish to understand their own unique body, emotions, mind, spirit dynamic. The workshops take participants into their interior being, where authentic and respectful healing energies create whatever change, experience, vision or release they require at that time. Contact the school for details if you would like to attend or sponsor workshops in your area. Seminars in Iridology, Herbal Medicine and Naturopathy are also offered throughout the year in Malaysia, Australia, Canada, India, the U.K. and Colorado every August.

Summer Schools

A month of full–time education is held throughout August in Boulder, Colorado, U.S.A. These seminars present the entire system of natural medicine, including Iridology, Naturopathy and Herbology, with special workshops in Elemental Energetics, an in–depth study of the elements of life that make up our body and our world, and clinical training. Send for a brochure for full details, dates and fees. The classes also include herbal apprentice training with expert wilderness, wildcrafting and herbal teachers, and hands–on training in the Herbs of Grace pharmacy and dispensary. Other classes and field trips take us into successful herbal companies, herb gardens, the University of Colorado Herbarium and the Herb Research Foundation.

Transformational Journeys

The school organizes a three–week trip every year to the Institute of Naturopathic and Yogic Sciences in Bangalore, India, which gives participants the benefit of experiencing a personal purification and regeneration treatment while they study naturopathy. Clients, students or others who would like to participate in a healing journey are welcome to contact the school to find out information about the next trip. The cost is approximately $1,000.00 plus the airfare of about $1,500.00. This study experience fulfills the requirement for the Naturopathy Diploma (ND).

Clinic

The school offers educational consultations to guide clients to become independently healthy. Telephone (303) 443–4882 for further information.

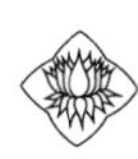

School of Natural Medicine Application Form

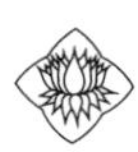

HOME STUDY COURSES – PAYMENT IN FULL

Iridology and the Foundation of Natural Medicine home study course.......... $400.00
Herbal Medicine home study course.......... $400.00
Naturopathy home study course.......... $300.00
Natural Physician – all 3 home courses – **BEST DISCOUNT!** $999.00

HOME STUDY COURSES –TIME PAYMENTS

Iridology & Foundation of Natural Medicine – 2 payments each of $225 – total $450..........$225.00
Herbal Medicine – 2 payments each of $225 – total $450.......... $225.00
Naturopathy – 2 payments each of $175 – total $350.......... $175.00
Natural Physician – 3 payments for 3 courses – 1st payment $400, 2nd and 3rd $325.......... $400.00

FOREIGN STUDENTS AIR MAIL SUPPLEMENTS

Canadian or Carribean students – per course add $15, 3 courses at once $40.......... $..........
International students – per course add $25 – Nat. Phys. 3 courses at once $65 .... $..........

SAMPLE LESSONS – each $20 US, $23 Canada, $27 international airmail.......... $..........

SUMMER SCHOOL – FOUNDATION OR CLINICAL TRAINING – 1 or 2 WEEKS

Deposit $200 for each week. Payment in Full $500 for each week .... $..........

SUMMER SCHOOL – WILDCRAFTING & ADVANCED HERBAL WEEKS – 1 or 2 weeks

Two weeks payment in full: $750. Deposit: $300 for 2 week session..........$..........
Individual week is $400 per week payment in full, Deposit $200 per week.......... $..........

SUMMER SCHOOL – Four weeks Foundation, Wildcrafting, Herbal & Clinical Training
SAVINGS – $1800 value for $1600, Deposit $500, Balance $1150.......... $..........

COMPLETE PACKAGE – 3 HOME COURSES AND FOUR–WEEK SUMMER SCHOOL
$2900 value – $2400 paid in full, Deposit $800 + $825 + $825 payment..........$..........

BOOKS, CASSETTES, SLIDES

Book rate postage, packing and insurance is included for the USA. Airmail extra.

IRIDOLOGY – *a complete guide to diagnosis & treatment*, hardback, $46 + post, packing..........$52.00
Herbs of Grace – *Becoming Independently Healthy*, 1993 revised patient workbook.......... $28.00
Iridology Coloring Book – Safi & Sharan, learn by coloring beautiful iris drawings.......... $22.00
Dictionary of Iridology – Safi's visual reference of Sharan's Iridology course.......... $23.00
Creative Menopause – *Illuminating Women's Health & Spirituality* 160 p, illustrations.......... $22.00
Creative Menopause – cassette, $12 + postage, packing..........$16.00
Elemental Energetics Music, cassettes – 5 tapes $66.00
Lectures in Copenhagen and Alternative Medicine Exhibition in London cassette..........$14.00
Slide Set – 15 color 35 mm slides with matching iris drawings to color, and case histories.......... $45.00

EXTRA POSTAGE FOR CANADA & INTERNATIONAL AIR MAIL:

Canada: add $4 for each book, $8 for IRIDOLOGY book, and $2 for each cassette..........$.........
International airmail: add $12 for each book, $20 for IRIDOLOGY book, and $5 for each cassette.

TOTAL PAYMENT .... $.........

Checks or money orders in U.S. $ only, payable to School of Natural Medicine.
Telephone, fax or write for Visa/MC, or fill in the form, fax, or mail with payment.

VISA/MASTERCHARGE # .... EXPIRATION DATE ....

NAME ....DATE ....

ADDRESS ....

.... Zip code .... Country .... Tel ....

SIGNATURE .... TOTAL PAYMENT $ ....

SCHOOL OF NATURAL MEDICINE, P. O. BOX 7369, BOULDER, CO 80306–7369, USA
Phone / FAX 303–443–4882